Applied
Anatomy & Physiology
Workbook

Brian R. Shmaefsky, PhD

Kingwood College
Kingwood, Texas

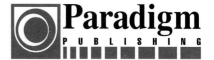

Senior Developmental Editor	Sonja Brown
Project Editor	Courtney Kost
Developmental Editor	Nadia Bidwell, Barking Dog Editorial
Content Expert	Melissa Curfman-Falvey
Cover and Text Designer	Leslie Anderson
Desktop Production	Leslie Anderson, Petrina Nyhan
Illustrator	Graphic World
Copy Editor	Colleen Duffy
Proofreader	Kay Savoie

Reviewers—The author and publisher wish to thank the following instructors and professionals for their valuable suggestions during the development of this book.

- Jerri Adler, BA, AA, CMA, CMT; Instructor (retired), Family and Health Careers Department, Lane Community College, Eugene, Oregon

- Robert Spears, PhD, Assistant Professor, Director of Undergraduate Research, Department of Biomedical Sciences, Baylor College of Dentistry-Texas A&M University System Health Science Center, Dallas, Texas

Publishing Team—Robert Cassel, Publisher; Janice Johnson, Vice President, Marketing; Lori Landwer, Marketing Manager; Shelley Clubb, Electronic Design and Production Manager.

Care has been taken to verify the accuracy of information presented in this book. The author, editors, and publisher, however, cannot accept any responsibility for errors or omissions or for consequences from application of the information in this book and make no warranty, expressed or implied, with respect to its content.

Text: ISBN 0-7638-2337-6
Text + Encore CD: ISBN 0-7638-2339-2

Care has been taken to verify the accuracy of information presented in this book. The author, editors, and publisher, however, cannot accept any responsibility for errors or omissions or for consequences from application of the information in this book and make no warranty, expressed or implied, with respect to its content.

Trademarks
Some of the pharmaceutical product names used in this book have been used for identification purposes only and may be trademarks or registered trademarks of their respective manufacturers.

TABLE OF CONTENTS

TABLE OF CONTENTS

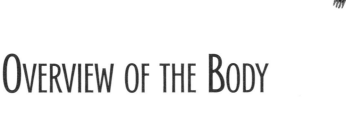

OVERVIEW OF THE BODY

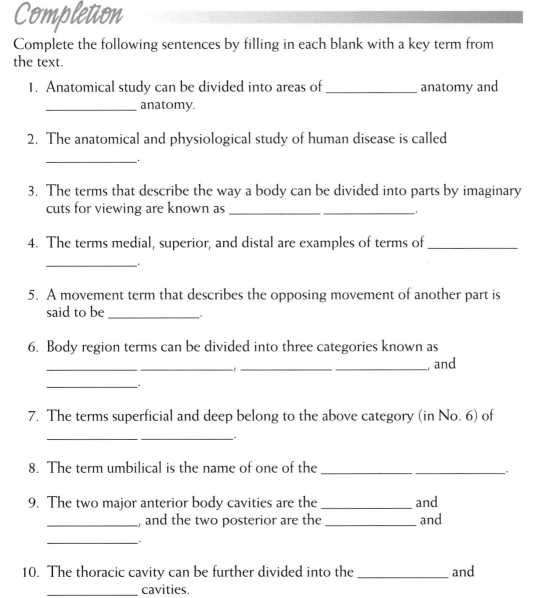

Completion

Complete the following sentences by filling in each blank with a key term from the text.

1. Anatomical study can be divided into areas of _____ anatomy and _____ anatomy.

2. The anatomical and physiological study of human disease is called _____.

3. The terms that describe the way a body can be divided into parts by imaginary cuts for viewing are known as _____ _____.

4. The terms medial, superior, and distal are examples of terms of _____ _____.

5. A movement term that describes the opposing movement of another part is said to be _____.

6. Body region terms can be divided into three categories known as _____ _____, _____ _____, and _____.

7. The terms superficial and deep belong to the above category (in No. 6) of _____ _____.

8. The term umbilical is the name of one of the _____ _____.

9. The two major anterior body cavities are the _____ and _____, and the two posterior are the _____ and _____.

10. The thoracic cavity can be further divided into the _____ and _____ cavities.

1

Matching

Match each of the following terms with the clue that best describes it by placing the letter of the term in the blank next to the correct clue.

a) lying on the back

b) movement away from the body

c) often used in place of the term "anatomy"

d) farther from the point of attachment

e) beneath or lower than

f) creates left and right sections

g) refers to the outer layer or surface covering

h) located on both sides of the body

i) surrounding the heart

j) body region named for its location above

k) the stomach

_____ abduction

_____ bilateral

_____ distal

_____ epigastric

_____ inferior

_____ morphology

_____ parietal

_____ pericardial

_____ sagittal plane

_____ supine

_____ abdominal

Complete the Terms Table

Complete the missing key terms and/or definitions in the following table.

Term	Definition
	anatomical and physiological study of human growth
cephalic	
	farther from the midline
	creation of superior and inferior sections
extension	
visceral	
	clinical body position with patient supine and legs bent
	body cavity containing the heart and lungs
	spinal column region of the neck
peritoneum	

Label the Graphic

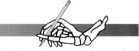

Identify each of the following terms in the illustration below. Write the number of the anatomy part on the line pointing to its location.

1. superior
2. inferior
3. medial
4. lateral
5. proximal
6. distal
7. anterior
8. posterior

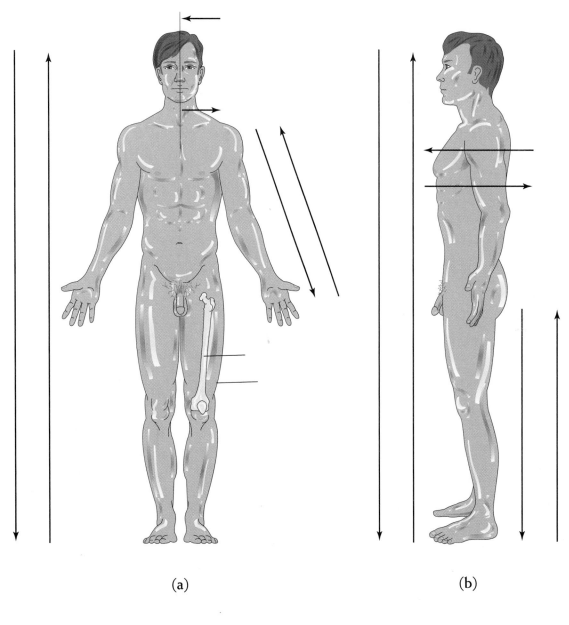

(a)   (b)

1. Which term best describes the location of the eyebrows with respect to the eyes?

2. Where are the toes in comparison to the knees?

3. The elbow is _____ to the wrist.

4. In relation to the sternum (breastbone), which term describes the location of the arms?

5. In anatomical position, which term locates the little finger in relation to the thumb?

6. What term describes the view of the body in Figure A?

7. Where is the chin is relation to the mouth?

8. If Figure A were turned in the opposite direction, which view of the body would be seen?

Color the Graphic

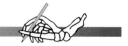

Color this illustration using the following color key:

cranial – blue
spinal – yellow
thoracic – red
abdominal – green
pelvic – purple

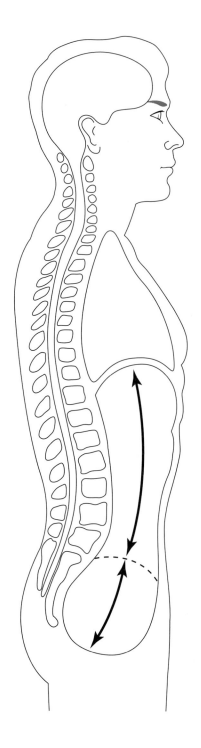

Practical Application

Write brief responses to the following scenarios.

1. List the parts of the hand that would be described by different directional orientation terms if the subject were standing with the palms flat against the legs rather than in standard anatomical position.

2. Identify five body parts or organs that are bilaterally located.

3. Name a clinical body position that might be used for each of the following medical situations:

   a) spinal adjustment

   b) gynecological exam

   c) dental examination of the upper jaw

   d) blood-pressure measurement

   e) abdominal surgery

4. Apply directional plane terms to each of the following descriptions:

   a) slicing a carrot in coin-like sections

b) cutting a pineapple perfectly in half so that each portion contains the stem

c) cutting a pickle into many thin lengthwise (longitudinal) slices

d) sawing a bed in two so that the headboard is separated from the footboard

5. Identify the body movement term involved in each of the following activities:
   a) "squat" exercises

   b) jumping jacks

   c) "pigeon-toe" placement of the feet

6. In which abdominopelvic quadrant might a patient with cirrhosis (inflammation of the liver) experience observable swelling?

   Which abdominopelvic region(s)?

7. Would it be correct to use abdominopelvic region terms to describe pain associated with the heart? Why or why not?

8. Which of the body cavities are connected? Explain.

9. In which major body cavity do you think the conditions called pleuritis and pericarditis would occur?

10. Name the spinal-column region with which each of the following items would have the most contact when worn:

a) belt

b) choker necklace

c) strapless bikini top

d) hip pockets

Crossword Puzzle

Complete the following crossword puzzle using key terms from the text.

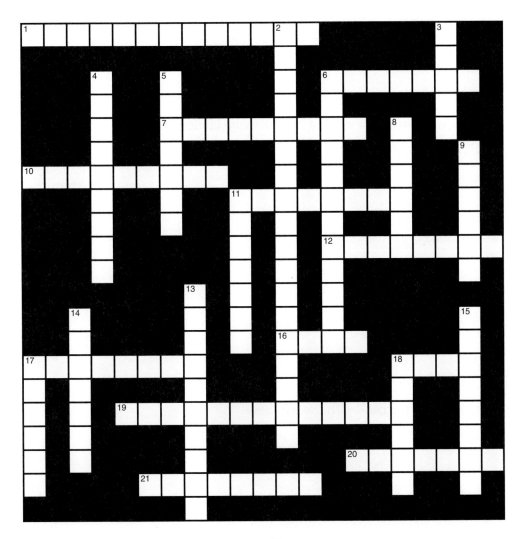

Across

1. supine body position
6. bending
7. arm or leg movement toward the body
10. hand or foot movement toward the body
11. head
12. closer to the point of attachment
16. away from the surface
17. membrane of the cranial and spinal cavity
18. left lateral clinical body position
19. superior lateral abdominopelvic region
20. sole of the foot
21. inferior lateral abdominopelvic region

Down

2. Abbr: location of the liver
3. face down
4. dorsal
5. cavity surrounding the brain
6. creates anterior and posterior sections
8. tailbone region
9. lower back
11. creates anterior and posterior sections
13. study of anatomical function
14. anterior or "belly" side
15. inner wall of an organ
17. closer to the midline
18. spinal region posterior to the pelvic bone

1. List the opposite directional orientation term for each of the following:

    a) inferior   _____

    b) medial   _____

    c) distal   _____

    d) posterior   _____

2. What is the name for each of the following clinical body positions?

    a) lying face down

    b) lying on the back

    c) sitting with the legs straight out, with the back supported

    d) lying on the back with the legs bent

    e) bending on the knees with the face down

3. Write the antagonist for each of the following body movements:

    a. extension

    b. abduction

    c. inversion

4. Name the four quadrants used in body-region terminology.

5. Name the nine abdominopelvic regions.

6. What is the difference between anatomy and physiology?

7. Define the term *directional plane*.

8. Observing a human tissue sample under a microscope would be an example of what division of anatomical study?

11

9. Describe proper anatomical position.

10. Anterior and posterior body sections are created by which kind of directional plane?

11. Distinguish between the terms *proximal* and *distal*.

12. What is the name given to the anatomical and physiological study of diseases?

13. Which type of plane creates equal-sized left and right halves?

14. Give an example of a flexion movement.

15. Use the correct term of directional orientation to describe the position of the arms in relation to the trunk of the body (in anatomical position).

16. Give an example of a superficial body structure.

17. List the two major anterior body cavities and their respective subdivisions.

18. List the posterior body cavities.

19. What does the parietal peritoneum touch?

20. Define the term *visceral*.

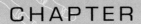

CHAPTER

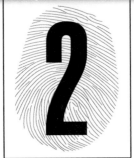

THE BODY'S CHEMICAL MAKEUP

Completion

Complete the following sentences by filling in each blank with a key term from the text.

1. The branch of natural science that deals with the composition of substances that make up a living organism's body structures, and their properties and reactions in body function is called _____ _____ or _____ _____.

2. The structure of each element consists of two major components called the atomic _____ and the atomic _____.

3. Two or more atoms joined together by chemical bonds form a _____.

4. Attached to the carbon skeleton of a biochemical is a _____ _____, which is responsible for its chemical activity.

5. Molecules that have the same _____ formula, but differ in their _____ formulas are called isomers.

6. The four organic chemical groups into which human molecules are categorized are _____, _____, _____, and _____ _____.

7. Lipids are commonly categorized into three groups: _____, _____, and _____.

8. Carbohydrates are classified as _____, _____, or _____ based on the number of "units" of which they are composed.

9. Small chains of amino acids form _____, and larger chains form _____.

10. A nucleotide has three parts: the _____ _____, _____ _____, and a _____ _____ _____.

Matching

Match each of the following terms with the clue that best describes it by placing the letter of the term in the blank next to the correct clue.

a) atomic number   _____ primary fat stored in the human body

b) atomic mass   _____ building block of nucleic acids

c) element   _____ 3-D structure of a protein

d) glycemic index   _____ sum of the number of protons and neutrons

e) hydrophilic   _____ cannot be chemically broken down

f) nucleotide   _____ containing the chemical carbon

g) organic   _____ water soluble

h) terpenoids   _____ category of fat in which vitamins belong

i) tertiary   _____ measure of available glucose in food

j) triglyceride   _____ number of protons in the nucleus

Complete the Terms Table

Complete the missing key terms and/or definitions in the following table.

Term	Definition
	anatomical and physiological study of human elements that have the same number of protons but differ in neutron number
ion	
	anything that has mass and occupies space
	an alcohol functional group
buffer	
monomer	
	having a stronger negative or positive charge on one side
	a fatty acid lacking hydrogen atoms and possessing double bonds
hydrogenate	
	a form of glucose stored in the liver and muscles
free-radical	
	the aging process of an organism

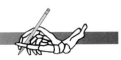
Identify each of the following terms in the illustration below.

1. Identify the type of chemical bond represented in each of the two illustrations below by writing the correct term, either **ionic** or **covalent**, beneath each picture.
2. Using the Periodic Table in Figure 2.2 (page 35 of the text, if necessary), identify each atom shown by writing the symbol used to represent its elemental name in the space directly above it. (Hint: Notice that the number of protons is indicated by the letter P inside each atom.)
3. In the ionic bond, indicate the ionic charge present on each of the atoms after bonding. (Hint: which subatomic part has changed in number for each atom, and how does it affect the electrical charge present on the atom?) The ionic charge should be written directly beneath each atom.

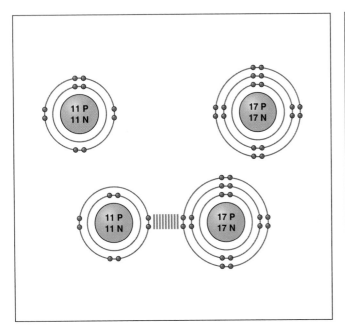

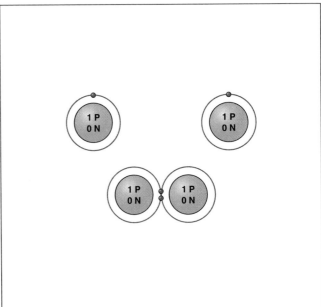

1. What is the atomic mass of the Na atom illustrated above?

2. How many electrons are in the outer orbital of each atom after ionic bonding?

3. Which subatomic particle is absent in the H atoms illustrated? Does this have any affect on their electrical charge?

4. Are the H atoms ions? Explain.

Color the Graphic

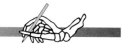

Color this illustration using the following color key:

electrons – purple
protons – red
neutrons – green
atomic nucleus – circle in blue
atomic orbitals – highlight in yellow

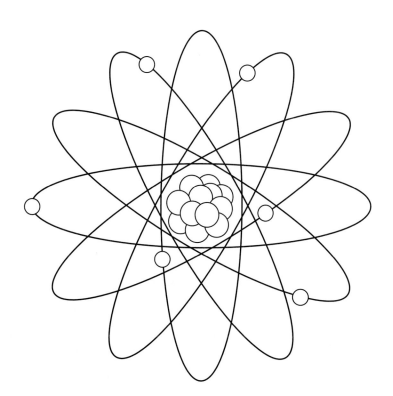

Practical Application

Write brief responses to the following scenarios.

1a. Hydrogen is the first element on the periodic table, and it has an atomic number of 1.008. What information does this give about each subatomic part?

1b. What additional information is obtained about subatomic ——————— by knowing the atomic mass?

2. The atomic weight of an element is the average of all possible isotopes (considering the naturally occurring proportion of each isotope). The atomic weight of hydrogen is 1.008. Which isotope of hydrogen, ^1H, ^2H, or ^3H, do you think is most abundant in nature? Explain why.

3. If a chemical reaction is defined as the interaction between two or more substances to form a new product, does adding the salt, NaCl, to water result in a chemical reaction? Why or why not?

4. If grapefruit juice has a pH of 3.0 and egg whites have a pH of 8.0, which contains more H^+ and, comparably, how many more?

5. Imagine that you are a research and development scientist working for a food manufacturing company. To create a new product, you need to use a fat that contains short carbon chains and is low in saturation. You have three frozen containers of lard, butter, and unhydrogenated vegetable oil, but the labels have fallen off, and you do not know which container holds which fat. Think of a simple way to choose the one to use. (You cannot rely on color, smell, or taste.)

6. A friend of yours decides to start taking a multivitamin. She assumes that more is better, so she increases the dosage to three tablets per day, rather than the manufacturer-recommended dose of one per day. What advice could you give her?

7. Would it be accurate to say that all carbohydrates containing glucose can supply that molecule as an energy source for the body? Explain.

8. Many digestive enzymes are made in the pancreas and sent to the small intestine where they act to break down food molecules. The stomach has a very low pH compared with the intestine and precedes the intestine in the digestive tract. If the pancreas were unable to produce digestive enzymes, would it be possible to ingest pancreatic enzymes and still maintain the same level of digestion? Explain.

9. Since most people know that humans need oxygen to survive, they might conclude that it is always "good" for the body. Respond to this idea given what you have learned about the factors involved in senescence.

10. Do you think it would be beneficial to add antioxidants to sunscreen to increase its effectiveness in decreasing sun damage?

Crossword Puzzle

Complete the following crossword puzzle using key terms from the text.

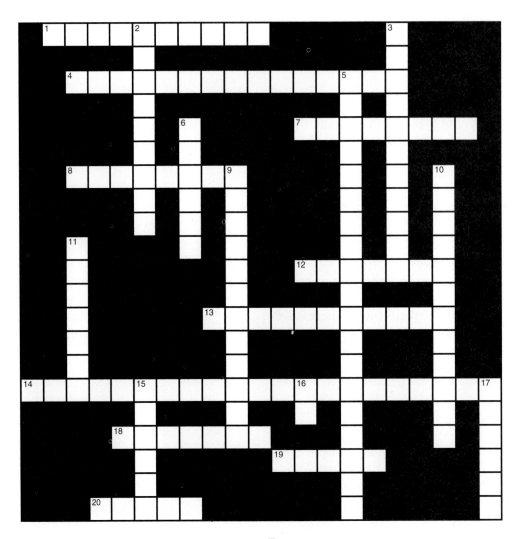

Across

1. "fat-loving"
4. Abbr: nucleotide containing ribose
7. organic acid group
8. basic
12. adenine and guanine
13. physiological balance or stability
14. Abbr: the most common energy transfer molecule
18. sugar with five carbons
19. type of organic compound usually insoluble in water
20. secondary protein structure

Down

2. functional group containing phosphorus
3. synonym for fatty acid
5. practiced by some athletes prior to an endurance event
6. describes mirror image isomers
9. ions that conduct electricity in water
10. glucose, fructose, galactose, and mannose
11. starch
15. cholesterol and sex hormones are examples
16. measure of H+ concentration in water
17. a type of functional protein

1. Organic chemistry is the study of chemicals that:
   a. only occur naturally
   b. are only found in living organisms
   c. contain the element carbon
   d. All of the above

2. An atom is:
   a. the smallest portion of an element that still retains its properties
   b. composed of subatomic particles
   c. consists of a nucleus surrounded by orbitals
   d. All of the above

3. The hydroxyl group:
   a. is chemically shown as OH
   b. helps molecules dissolve in water
   c. is also known as an alcohol group
   d. All of the above

4. Molecules that have the same chemical formula, but that differ in structural formula are:
   a. always similar in their physical and chemical properties
   b. called isomers
   c. cannot be classified as biochemicals
   d. All of the above

5. A common functional group containing nitrogen is called the:
   a. carboxyl group
   b. carbonyl group
   c. sulfate group
   d. amino group

6. Acids are:
   a. electron acceptors
   b. lower than 7.0 on the pH scale
   c. chemically shown as OH
   d. All of the above

7. Which of the following terms are best matched?
   a. fat soluble/hydrophilic
   b. fat insoluble/hydrophobic
   c. fat soluble/lipophobic
   d. fat insoluble/lipophobic

8. Cholesterol is a:
   a. protein
   b. nucleic acid
   c. carbohydrate
   d. lipid

9. Which of the following terms are best matched?
   a. monomer nucleotide/RNA
   b. polymer nucleotide/ATP
   c. polymer nucleotide/DNA
   d. All of the above

10. Choose the pair of terms that correctly complete the following sentence:
    Single units of carbohydrates are joined by _____ bonds to
    form polysaccharides, while amino acids are linked by _____
    bonds to form polypeptides.
    a. ionic/protein
    b. chiral/nucleotide
    c. glycosidic/peptide
    d. All of the above

11. Which one of the three categories of lipids is most abundant in the body?
    a. terpenoids
    b. sterols
    c. glycerides
    d. All are contained in similar amounts

12. Which of the following is not a monosaccharide?
    a. glucose
    b. maltose
    c. fructose
    d. galactose

13. Nucleotide monomers are involved in:
    a. determining genetic traits
    b. transferring energy
    c. making proteins
    d. All of the above

14. What product of carbohydrates and fats is most important for the body?
    a. energy
    b. amino acids
    c. structural material
    d. electrolytes

15. A diet lacking proper nutrition might cause:
    a. malnutrition
    b. undernutrition
    c. cravings
    d. All of the above

16. Which of the following best describes senescence?
    a. the process of body aging brought about by molecular decay
    b. the result, in part, of free radical oxidation
    c. the result, in part, of the effects of ultraviolet radiation
    d. All of the above

17. List the subatomic parts contributing to each of the following:

    a. atomic number   _____   _____

    b. atomic mass   _____   _____

    c. atomic bonding   _____   _____

    d. isotopes   _____   _____

    e. ions   _____   _____

18. Match each protein level of organization with the letter of the term or phrase to which it is most related.

    a) 3-D arrangement   _____ primary structure

    b) linear amino-acid arrangement   _____ secondary structure

    c) helix or sheet   _____ tertiary structure

    d) two or more polypeptide chains _____ quaternary structure

19. List two sources of free radicals.

20. List four functions of fat in the body.

21. List four common disaccharides. Which common monosaccharide is present in all four?

22. Briefly explain what is meant by the polarity of an H_2O molecule.

23. Why are buffers important in the human body?

24. What is the difference between an element and a compound? Give an example of each. Would it be correct to say that they are both formed from molecules?

25. Why are covalent bonds the most common bonds in biochemicals?

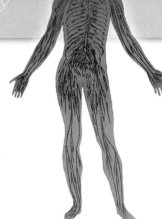

CHAPTER

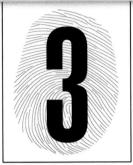

ORGANIZATION OF THE BODY

Completion

Complete the following sentences by filling in each blank with a key term from the text.

1. The physiological environment of a cell includes both the _____ and _____ environments.

2. If a molecule has gained an electron through a chemical reaction, it has been _____ , and if it has lost an electron, it has been _____ .

3. Chemical reactions that use up energy are called _____ , while those that release energy are _____ .

4. Movement of molecules across the cell membrane following the diffusion gradient is _____ transport, while movement going against the diffusion gradient is _____ transport.

5. A cell will gain water when it is in a _____ environment, and it will lose water when it is in a _____ environment.

6. The three divisions of cell structural components are the _____ _____ , the _____ , and the _____ .

7. Metabolic reactions that use energy to build body components are called _____ , while those that break down molecules to provide energy and raw materials needed for such activity are called _____ .

8. _____ takes place in the cytoplasm, but the remaining stages of aerobic respiration occur in the _____ .

9. Gene expression consists of two stages: _____ and _____ . _____ occurs in the nucleus, during which DNA is copied to create messenger ribonucleic acid (mRNA). _____ occurs in the cytoplasm on organelles called _____ and synthesizes _____ .

10. Sexual cell division is called meiosis. It occurs in two nuclear divisions: The first separates _____ chromosomes, and the second separates _____ .

11. The four types major types of human tissue are _____ , _____ , _____ , and _____ .

12. _____ glands, which release their secretions into the blood, and _____ glands, whose secretions travel through ducts to particular body locations, are both composed of _____ cells.

13. Connective tissue can be classified as _____ , such as blood, or _____ , such as bone, _____ , _____ , and tendons.

14. The three types of muscle tissue are _____ , _____ , and _____ .

15. _____ is a decrease in the size of a cell, tissue, or organ, while the enlargement of these body components is known as _____ .

16. The telomeres, or chromosome ends, of cancer cells do not undergo shortening following _____ (cell division), thus, enabling them to be immortal.

Matching

Match each of the following terms with the clue that best describes it by placing the letter of the term in the blank next to the correct clue.

a) anaphase

b) blood

c) calorie

d) chromatid

e) codon

f) epithelium

g) fatty change

h) gamete

_____ stage of karyokinesis during which chromosomes separate

_____ the "outcome" of a chemical reaction

_____ cells working together to perform a special function

_____ standard unit of heat

_____ type of exocytosis

_____ lack organelles and possess nucleoid genome

_____ sum of all chemical reactions in the body

_____ process driven by the electron transport chain to produce ATP

i) lymphatic   _____ three nucleotides coding for a specific amino acid

j) metabolism   _____ egg or sperm

k) necrosis   _____ multilayered

l) neuroglia   _____ tissue that forms a lining or covering in the body

m) oxidative phosphorylation   _____ connective-tissue type

n) product   _____ voluntary muscle tissue

o) prokaryotic   _____ nervous tissue cell

p) skeletal   _____ body system that fights disease

q) secretion   _____ localized tissue death

r) stratified   _____ can occur from excessive alcohol intake

s) telomere   _____ a copy of a chromosome

Complete the Terms Table

Complete the missing key terms and/or definitions in the following table.

Term	Definition
	anatomical and physiological study of human growth
cell	
	substance that dissolves other chemicals
organ	
substrate	
	passive transport process that utilizes carrier proteins to move molecules across a semipermeable membrane
	the potential of water to move across a selectively permeable membrane
heredity	
	a strand of DNA that actually codes for genes
somatic cells	
haploid	
amyloid	
	an embryological germ layer that forms bone and muscle
	cells that do not undergo differentiation into embryological germ layers, but retain their ability to differentiate
pseudostratified	
	a condition in which diseased cells move from one location to another, continuing their abnormal function at the new site

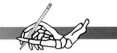

Label the Graphic

Identify each of the following terms in the illustration below. Write the number of the anatomical part on the line pointing to its location.

1. transcription
2. translation

Place the number for each of the following terms on the line next to where each is represented on the illustration:

3. gene
4. pre-mRNA
5. processed RNA (at two locations)
6. protein
7. ribosome
8. RNA

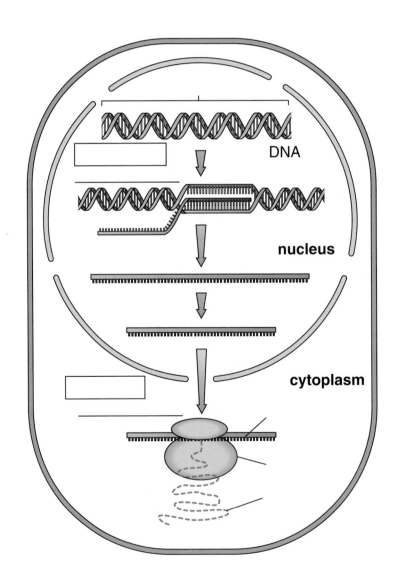

Color the Graphic

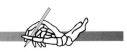

Color this illustration using the following color key:

cytoplasm – yellow
DNA – black
Golgi apparatus – dark green
lysosome – grey
mitochondrion – orange
nuclear membrane – brown
nucleolus – dark blue
nucleus – light blue
ribosomes – red
RNA – white
rough endoplasmic reticulum – light green
smooth endoplasmic reticulum – pink

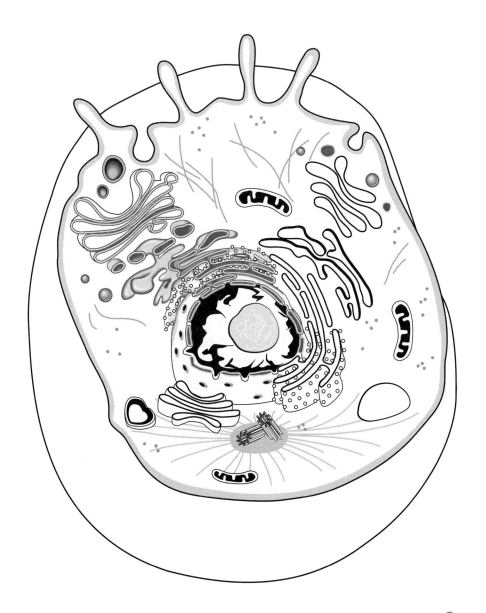

Practical Application

Write brief responses to the following scenarios.

1. Do unicelluar organisms, such as bacteria and yeast cells, exhibit differentiation? Explain.

2. Why is water such an ideal substance for the body's physiological environment?

3. In terms of energy conversion, how is the energy needed by a weight lifter created, and what type of energy does his/her activity create?

4. What do you think would happen to an individual's red blood cells if the osmolarity of the plasma (liquid portion of the blood) was altered by continuous intravenous administration of pure water (containing no electrolytes).

5. The text states that "Today it is accepted that not all organisms have a cell as the basic unit of structure." Give examples of one such organism that is considered to be "living," and apply what you have learned about cell structure to substantiate why it does not have true cells.

6. Do you think that an individual's body would be undergoing more anabolic metabolism or more catabolic metabolism following a meal high in carbohydrates? Briefly explain.

7. A common form of Down's syndrome (a disease that is predestined at conception that results in physical anomalies and mental retardation) is caused by a genetic defect called trisomy. In this disease, a particular chromosome in the affected individual's genome is present in triplicate, rather than in the diploid (paired) state of normal chromosomes. This means that either the egg or the sperm creating the offspring carried a diploid number of chromosome 21, rather than the normal haploid number of chromosomes in a gamete. Use your knowledge of cell division to determine which type would cause the genetic defect to occur, and at what particular stage of division.

8. A lab technician prepared slides of tissue samples and forgot to label their source in the body. Samples had been taken from a patient's heart wall and the stomach wall. What visual clues might help differentiate the two samples?

9. How could one distinguish between dysplasia and hyperplasia?

10. When asked about the role that telomeres play in cellular aging, a student replies that this part of the chromosome makes proteins that initiate cellular death. Respond to the accuracy of this statement.

Crossword Puzzle

Complete the following crossword puzzle using key terms from the text.

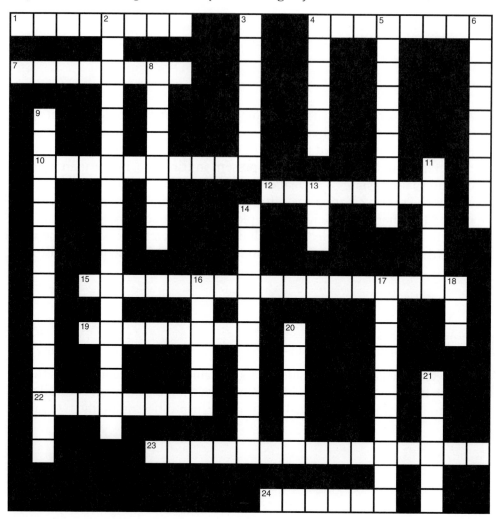

Across

1. connective-tissue protein
4. flat-shaped epithelial cells
7. highest level of hierarchical organization
10. cell excretion is an example
12. property of water that reduces its evaporation and limits dehydration
15. created by unequal intracellular and extracellular solutions
19. type of procaryote
22. stimulate cell division
23. allows for physiological specialization of cells
24. dissolved substance in a solution

Down

2. requires oxygen to produce energy from food
3. "reduction" cell division to produce gametes
4. muscle tissue of blood vessels
5. programmed cell death
6. molecular "building"
8. gene alteration
9. product of pyruvic acid oxidation
11. not cancerous
13. Abbr: type of regulatory DNA
14. a food calorie
16. water-lubricating fluid
17. cell cycle stage of chromosome duplication
18. Abbr: Krebs cycle
20. organic catalyst
21. positive ion

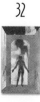

1. The level of human organizational hierarchy that is above the cellular level is the:

   a) molecular level
   b) organ level
   c) tissue level
   d) envirome level

2. Conditions that influence homeostasis of the aqueous environment of cells are determined by:

   a) pH
   b) chemical reactions
   c) molecular transport across the membrane
   d) All of the above

3. Which pair of terms most accurately completes the following sentence: *Food is a form of _____ energy, which provides the ability for muscle movement, which is a form of _____ energy?*

   a) electrical/mechanical
   b) thermal/kinetic
   c) chemical/potential
   d) potential/kinetic

4. In the chemical reactions of aerobic respiration, what molecule is the initial substrate?

   a) acetyl coA
   b) glucose
   c) pyruvic acid
   d) starch

5. Which waste product produced in large amounts by a diet high in protein and low in carbohydrate content can lead to dehydration in the body?

   a) glycerol
   b) carboxyl
   c) urea
   d) amino acids

6. The region of an enzyme that is the point of its attachment to another molecule is called the:

   a) amine bond
   b) protein activator
   c) ionization point
   d) active site

7. If the content of nitrogen in a cell's environment is isotonic to the cell's interior, this means that:

   a) there is no movement of nitrogen into or out of body cells
   b) nitrogen will travel across the cell membrane in both directions at a similar rate
   c) there is more nitrogen in the air than in the cell's interior
   d) there is less nitrogen in air than in the cell's interior

8. Facilitated diffusion requires the use of:

   a) active transport
   b) osmosis
   c) carrier proteins
   d) All of the above

9. Excretion and secretion are examples of:

   a) diffusion
   b) active transport pumping
   c) passive transport
   d) bulk active transporter

10. The human body is:

    a) composed of eucaryotic cells
    b) described as unicellular
    c) composed of procaryotic cells
    d) All of the above

11. Proteins in the cell membrane:

    a) help provide cell communication
    b) can be involved in molecular transport
    c) aid in cell adhesion
    d) All of the above

12. Which of the following describes a correct order related to aerobic respiration?

    a) glycolysis → Krebs cycle → fermentation
    b) electron transport chain → Krebs cycle → glycolysis
    c) fermentation → glycolysis → Krebs cycle
    d) glycolysis → Krebs cycle → electron transport chain

13. In gene expression, transcribed DNA would be best described as:

    a) a gene
    b) polypeptide
    c) mRNA
    d) translated DNA

14. Which of the following terms is not one of the four major human tissue types:

    a) glandular
    b) epithelial
    c) connective
    d) nervous

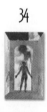

15. Epithelial tissues are categorized by:

   a) shape and size
   b) layering and shape
   c) number of nuclei
   d) All of the above

16. Match each type of cell division with the letter(s) of all the terms pertaining
    to it:

   mitosis: _____

   meiosis: _____

   a) gamete formation
   b) somatic cells
   c) haploid products
   d) diploid products
   e) asexual reproduction
   f) sexual reproduction

17. Match each term of the cell cycle with the clue it matches best:

   a) DNA replication   _____ anaphase

   b) equatorial plane   _____ cytokinesis

   c) differentiation   _____ G_0

   d) chromatid or chromosome   _____ interphase
      separation

   e) spindle fiber formation   _____ metaphase

   f) cytoplasmic division   _____ prophase

18. Match each of the following terms with the letter of the most appropriate
    clue:

   a. increase in cell size   _____ amyloid deposition

   b. abnormal growth pattern   _____ atrophy

   c. decrease in cell size   _____ dysplasia

   d. Alzheimer's disease   _____ hyperplasia

   e. increase in cell number   _____ hypertrophy

19. In respect to the hierarchy of human structure, arrange the following terms
    in order from lowest to highest: atom, body systems, cell, molecule, organ-
    ism, organ, society, and tissue.

20. What roles do ions play in the body's physiological environment, and how can they be lost from the body?

21. List the parts of a cell that are interrelated by their function of producing and transporting molecules and/or cell parts.

22. The body's physiological environment can be described as a mixture, or _____, composed of water, which is the _____ portion, and the _____ component, which comprises the dissolved biochemicals.

23. The three types of muscle tissue are known as _____, _____, and _____.

24. Connective tissue types are classified as either _____ or _____.

25. Because they lack the ability to undergo mitosis, fat-, skeletal-, and nervous-tissue cells are subject to damage in the cytoplasm, which is called _____ _____ _____.

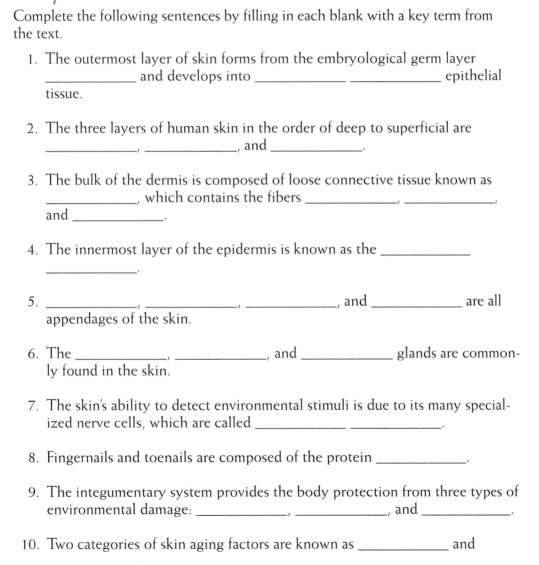

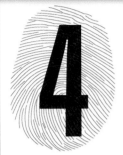

THE SKIN AND ITS PARTS

Completion

Complete the following sentences by filling in each blank with a key term from the text.

1. The outermost layer of skin forms from the embryological germ layer _____ and develops into _____ _____ epithelial tissue.

2. The three layers of human skin in the order of deep to superficial are _____, _____, and _____.

3. The bulk of the dermis is composed of loose connective tissue known as _____, which contains the fibers _____, _____, and _____.

4. The innermost layer of the epidermis is known as the _____ _____.

5. _____, _____, _____, and _____ are all appendages of the skin.

6. The _____, _____, and _____ glands are commonly found in the skin.

7. The skin's ability to detect environmental stimuli is due to its many specialized nerve cells, which are called _____ _____.

8. Fingernails and toenails are composed of the protein _____.

9. The integumentary system provides the body protection from three types of environmental damage: _____, _____, and _____.

10. Two categories of skin aging factors are known as _____ and _____.

37

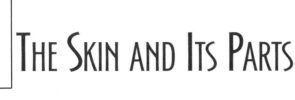

Matching

Match each of the following terms with the clue that best describes it by placing the letter of the term in the blank next to the correct clue.

a) commensals   _____ inborn

b) furuncle   _____ associated with thick skin

c) hair medulla   _____ skin and hair "oil"

d) hair papilla   _____ outermost epidermal layer

e) inherent   _____ white "half-moon" portion of the fingernail

f) lipoma   _____ hair follicle base

g) lunula   _____ inner layer of hair

h) sebum   _____ beneficial skin bacteria

i) stratum corneum   _____ fat-cell tumor

j) stratum lucidum   _____ inflammation of hair follicles

k) tinea   _____ condition of hypopigmention

l) vitiligo   _____ ringworm

Complete the Terms Table

Complete the missing key terms and/or definitions in the following table.

Term	Definition
	anatomical and physiological study of human growth
angiogenic factor	
malpighian layer	
	layer of epidermis that contains immune system cells
	inflammation of the fibrous connective tissue of the subcutaneous layer of skin
pheromones	
	pain-sensing structures that are distributed throughout the lower part of the epidermis
	touch receptors found in the mucus membranes of the mouth
arrector pili muscle	
	nerve cells that convert environmental stimuli into body signals
	burn category that characterizes reparable damage of the stratum spinosum and stratum generativum layers of the epidermis
solar lentigenes	
	group of viruses that cause warts in humans

Label the Graphic

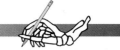

Identify each of the following terms in the illustration below. Write the number of the anatomical part on the line pointing to its location. One term will be used twice.

1. adipose tissue
2. collagen
3. dermal papilla
4. dermis
5. eccrine sweat gland
6. epidermis
7. hair follicle
8. malpighian layer (melanin layer)
9. opening of eccrine sweat gland
10. sebaceous gland
11. stratum corneum
12. stratum germinativum
13. subcutaneous layer

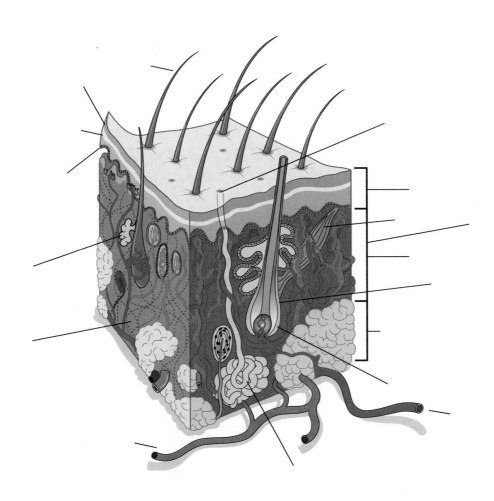

THE SKIN AND ITS PARTS

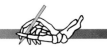

Color the Graphic

Color this illustration using the following color key:

adipose tissue (subcutaneous layer) – yellow
arrector pili muscle – purple
dermis – brown
epidermis – pink
hair bulb – red
hair follicle – orange
hair papilla – blue
hair shaft – black
sebaceous gland – green

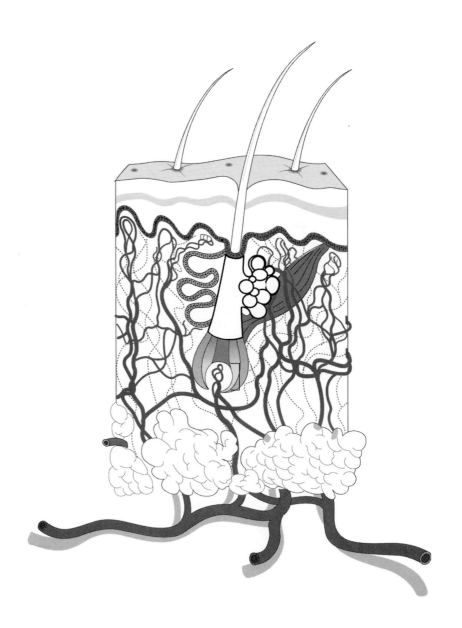

Practical Application

Write brief responses to the following scenarios.

1. A child asks you why his lips "turn blue" when it is cold outside. What would you explain to this child?

2. How might a lower-than-normal fibroblast cell population affect an individual's skin?

3. A person is sitting next to you in a steam room and inquires as to why it feels hotter in the steam room than it does in the dry sauna even though both areas are kept at the same temperature. How would you respond to this question?

4. A student has recently learned that pheromones are secreted by sweat glands. He wants to design a study to investigate whether or not certain animals seem to be affected by human pheromones. He plans to collect sweat from the headbands and gloves worn by individuals undergoing strenuous exercise to use in his study. Would you agree that this is a good plan?

5. A friend says that his family only uses soap and shampoo that have an anti-bacterial agent added. Explain to them why this might not be such a good idea.

6. A friend of yours is trying to lose weight and has started a diet that excessively restricts calories. She has also begun an extremely vigorous exercise program. She has noticed that her hair seems to be thinning, so has been brushing it excessively in hopes of stimulating its growth. What factors of her activity might be contributing to her noticeable hair loss?

7. Investigators often collect hair for forensic analysis. What types of clues can be obtained through hair analysis?

8. An entrepreneur is excited about his idea to develop a body lotion that totally prevents body sweating. Explain to him why it would not be advisable to pursue the development of this product.

9. If a third-degree burn results in irreparable damage to the deeper layers of skin where pain receptors are found, why do victims of severe burns experience pain?

10. A friend of yours has regularly used cosmetics to enhance her appearance. She has also always been adamant about following a cleansing regimen to remove her makeup, which is followed by the use of astringents and moisturizers. She often boasts that her meticulous skin care habits are much healthier than your more "natural" approach to beauty. Do you agree?

Crossword Puzzle

Complete the following crossword puzzle using key terms from the text.

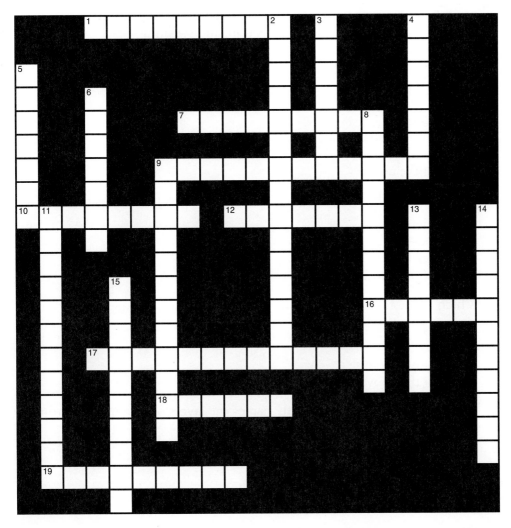

Across

1. environmental aging factors
7. increased production and inflammation of the skin cells
9. shedding of skin
10. rash caused by the bacterium *Staphyyloccus aureus*
12. chemical of skin pigmentation
16. fetal body hair
17. type of birthmark
18. adult body hair
19. sweat gland tumor

Down

2. beneficial fungus of the digestive and female reproductive tract
3. darkening of skin commonly associated with pregnancy
4. ear wax
5. ____'s Corpuscles: receptors of constant touch
6. arthropod that causes inflammation of the eyelashes
8. anti-aging treatment that promotes swelling of the skin
9. progressive tissue deterioration
11. special sensory nerves of the fingertips
13. genetic lack of pigmentation
14. collagen and elastin secreting cells
15. subcutaneous layer of skin

THE SKIN AND ITS PARTS

1. The four functions of skin in order of magnitude are:

    a) protection, waste excretion, sensation, and heat regulation
    b) sensation, heat regulation, protection, and sweating
    c) protection, respiration, heat regulation, and sensation
    d) protection, heat regulation, sensation, and waste excretion

2. Which of the following is an adaptive feature of skin?

    a) hair growth
    b) nail formation on the fingers and toes
    c) callus formation
    d) All of the above

3. From which of the embryological germ layers does the dermis develop?

    a) ectoderm
    b) mesoderm
    c) endoderm
    d) All of the above

4. Which of the following can contribute to hair loss?

    a) genes
    b) stress
    c) excessive exercise
    d) All of the above

5. Which of the following correctly names the layers of skin in order from superficial to deep?

    a) epidermis, dermis, hypodermis
    b) dermis, hypodermis, epidermis
    c) epidermis, endodermis, dermis
    d) hypodermis, dermis, epidermis

6. The dermal layer of skin contains:

    a) loose areolar connective tissue
    b) elastin, collagen, and reticular fibers
    c) skin appendages
    d) All of the above

7. Which of the following is not associated with the hypodermis or subcutaneous layer?

    a) keratin
    b) adipose
    c) fascia
    d) nerves

8. The area of the fingers and toes where nail growth takes place is called the:

    a) nail matrix
    b) lunula
    c) nail plate
    d) nail root

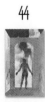

9. Which of the following best describes hair?

   a) modified stratum corneum
   b) a shaft composed of an inner medulla and an outer cortex
   c) "colored" by keratin and/or melanin
   d) All of the above

10. Which of the following word pairs describing human hair is correct:

   a) pubic : body hair
   b) vellus : fetal/infant hair
   c) terminal : head hair
   d) lanugo : genital hair

11. Mechanical damage to the skin in minimized by which of the following?

   a) callus formation
   b) microorganisms
   c) sebum production
   d) All of the above

12. Commensal organisms

   a) are undesirable for healthy skin.
   b) help keep disease-causing organisms from thriving on the skin.
   c) are not commonly found on healthy skin.
   d) All of the above

13. The skin functions to regulate body heat through which of the following?

   a) the control of blood flow in vessels
   b) evaporation of sweat
   c) adipose tissue insulation
   d) All of the above

14. Which of the following are the primary structures of waste excretion in the skin?

   a) eccrine sweat glands
   b) apocrine sweat glands
   c) sebaceous glands
   d) All of the above contribute equally

15. Third-degree burns

   a) involve only the superficial layers of the skin.
   b) are defined as damage to the stratum germinativum.
   c) usually heal through skin regeneration.
   d) commonly involve nerve cell loss in the dermis.

16. Skin cancer is which of the following?

   a) a degenerative skin disorder
   b) has an underlying genetic component
   c) is induced by sunlight or chemical exposure
   d) All of the above

17. The most common bacterial skin infections are caused by which of the following?

   a) dermatophytes
   b) *Candida albicans*
   c) *Staphylococcus aureus*
   d) All of the above

18. Which of the following best descrives skin aging?

   a) causes homeostasis disruption that contributes to overall body aging
   b) is due to both intrinsic and extrinsic factors
   c) is characterized by many gross anatomical changes
   d) All of the above

19. Match each of the following layers associated with the epidermis with the letter of the clue pertaining to it:

   a) generates upper layers   _____ dermal papilla layer

   b) connects epidermis to dermis   _____ malpighian layer

   c) contains immune cells   _____ stratum basale

   d) melanin deposition   _____ stratum compactum

   e) associated with thick skin   _____ stratum corneum

   f) desquamation   _____ stratum granulosum

   g) keratocyte origination   _____ stratum lucidum

   h) single layer of keratinized cells   _____ *statum spinosum*

20. Match the letter of each of the following skin sensory receptors with the clue pertaining to it:

   a) free nerve endings   _____ touch receptors found in the fingertips

   b) Krause's end bulbs   _____ pressure or constant touch

   c) Meissner's corpuscles   _____ pain sensory receptors

   d) Merkel cells   _____ deep tactile receptors of the hypodermis

   e) pacinian corpuscles   _____ tactile receptors in the dermal papilla

   f) Ruffini's receptors   _____ tactile receptors of the mouth

21. Match the letter of each of the following types of benign skin tumors with the clue that pertains to it:

   a) lipoma   _____ rough, greasy dark growth

   b) moles   _____ adipose tissue

   c) sebaceous hyperplasia   _____ pigmented squamous cells

   d) seborrheic keratosis   _____ sweat gland ducts

   e) syringomas   _____ oil glands

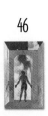

22. Name two accessory structures of hair and describe the function of each.

23. List the three types of glands commonly found in the skin and their respective secretions and body locations.

24. List the components of the integumentary system.

25. What benefit do cerumen and sebum have for the body?

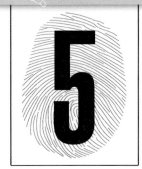

THE SKELETAL SYSTEM

Completion

Complete the following sentences by filling in each blank with a key term from the text.

1. The human skeleton is divided into two major groups: the _____ division and the _____ division.

2. The skull is composed of two groups of bones: _____ and _____ .

3. The sutures of the skull are the _____, _____, _____, and _____.

4. The five regions of the vertebral column are _____, _____, _____, _____, and _____.

5. The thoracic skeleton includes the _____, _____, _____, and _____.

6. Bones can be categorized into four types of shapes: _____, _____, _____, and _____.

7. A joint can be _____ classified into one of three types known as _____, _____, or _____; or it can be _____ classified as a _____, _____, or _____.

8. Human bones, except teeth, can be classified as either _____ or _____ .

9. The two types of bone marrow are _____, which contains fat cells, and _____, which contains _____ cells.

10. The two major types of embryological bone formation are _____ ossification and _____ ossification.

Matching

Match each of the following terms with the clue that best describes it by placing the letter of the term in the blank next to the correct clue.

a) articulation   _____ immovable joint

b) bursa   _____ bone cells

c) capitate   _____ ends of long bones

d) communited   _____ bone tissue building cells

e) epiphyses   _____ synovial fluid-filled sac

f) hyoid   _____ bone surface connective tissue

g) ossification   _____ arch-shaped bone under lower jaw

h) osteoblasts   _____ formed within a tendon

i) osteocytes   _____ the process of bone formation

j) palatine   _____ bone junction

k) patella   _____ fracture causing bone displacement

l) periostium   _____ articulates with tibia and fibula

m) sesamoid bone   _____ carpal bone

n) synarthrosis   _____ kneecap

o) talus   _____ roof of the mouth

Complete the Terms Table

Complete the missing key terms and/or definitions in the following table.

Term	Definition
wormian bones	
	main body of a long bone
	passageway for nerves and blood vessels from the periostium to the haversian canal
canaliculi	
	soft fat-cell tissue found within most bones
	cells that break down bone and cartilage during bone development and repair
rheumatoid arthritis	
fibromyalgia	
	socket of the pelvic girdle forming the articulation point with the femur
pubic symphysis	
	soft areas on the infant skull that are the result of incomplete development of the intramembranous bone
angulation	

Label the Graphic

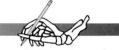

Identify each of the following terms in the illustration below. Write the number of the anatomical part on the line pointing to its location.

1. carpals
2. clavicle
3. cranium
4. femur
5. fibula
6. humerus
7. ilium
8. ischium
9. manubrium
10. metacarpals
11. patella
12. radius
13. pectoral (shoulder) girdle
14. pelvic girdle
15. phalanges
16. pubis
17. scapula
18. skull
19. sternum
20. tibia
21. ulna
22. vertebral column
23. xiphoid process

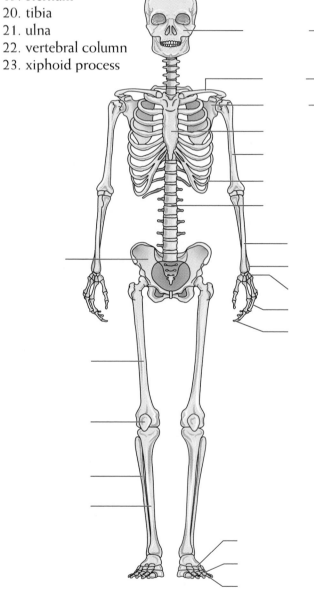

Color the Graphic

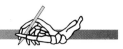

Color this illustration using the following color key:

frontal – yellow
lacrimal – purple
mandible – brown
maxilla – green
nasal – red
occipital – orange
parietal – light blue
sphenoid – dark blue
temporal – pink
zygomatic bone – white

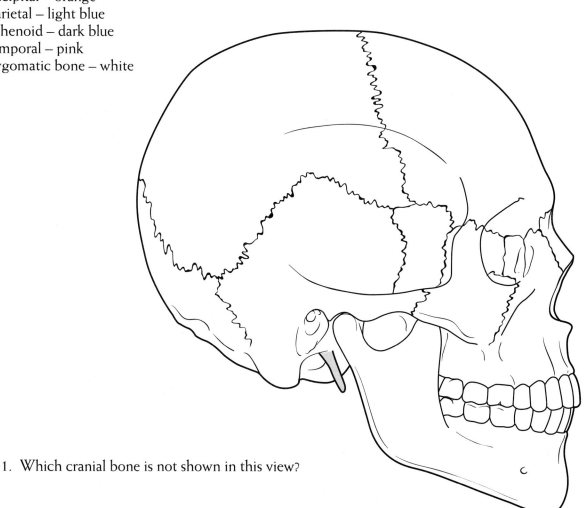

1. Which cranial bone is not shown in this view?

2. Which facial bones cannot be seen in this lateral view?

3. Name three important specialized temporal bone features that are visible in this lateral view.

51

Practical Application

Write brief responses to the following scenarios.

1. Describe which bones could be involved in a "broken nose."

2. Why does a broken clavicle cause restriction of head and arm movement?

3. Many people believe that the name "funny bone" (in reference to the elbow, especially when hit against a hard surface) is derived from an association with the name of the upper arm bone. What might be the reason for this word association, and is it really accurate?

4. Which bone in the forearm is located "thumbside?" Is it the lateral or medial of the two forearm bones when the body is in anatomical position? How does its position change in relation to the other bone of the forearm when the hands are in the position opposite of the true anatomical position?

5. Which bones and specific "structure" form the medial and lateral protrusions felt in the ankle area? Which bone of the foot is articulated with these bones to connect it to the leg?

6. What portion of the hands and feet has bones with one common name, and what terminology is used to differentiate each of these bones from one another? Give an example by naming the bone that forms the tip of the thumb and the bone that forms the middle of the middle toe.

7. List two specific areas of the body, and the specific features of each, that would help a forensic pathologist to identify the gender of a person from his/her skeletal remains.

8. When one thinks of the skeletal system, the anatomical arrangement of the bones is the predominant feature that comes to mind. What is limiting about this view in light of the fact that the the skeletal system is a true organ system that interacts with other body systems?

9. Can you think of a letter association that might help someone remember the names and respective functions of each of the cell types that begins with the root "osteo" and plays a role in endochondrial bone formation?

10. The text refers to stress fractures as breaks in bones that are too small to heal. Use the information in the textbook that deals with bone healing to explain why such small fractures may not heal.

Crossword Puzzle

Complete the following crossword puzzle using key terms from the text.

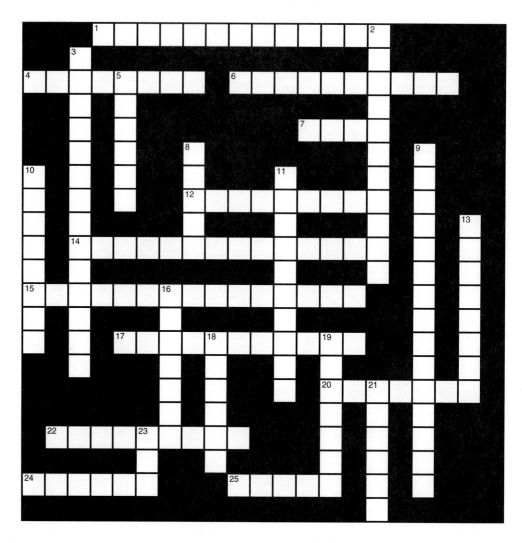

Across

1. skull opening for the spinal cord
4. forms bump on the wrist
6. bone fracture with break and bend of bone
7. build up of oxalic acid in joints
12. fingers or toes
14. center of osteon
15. area of active bone growth
17. slightly movable joint
20. wrist bones
22. process forming the elbow point
24. one of the tarsal bones
25. upper bone of pelvic girdle

Down

2. long foot bones
3. deterioration of articular cartilage at bone ends
5. lateral lower leg bone
8. connective tissue disease
9. filled with bone marrow
10. connects bone to bone
11. spongy bone
13. tooth socket
16. shoulder bone
18. connects muscle to bone
19. posterior lower bone of pelvic girdle
21. "thumbside" of the lower arm bone
23. immune stem cell bone marrow

1. Which of the following is true of the axial skeleton?
   a) includes the arms and legs
   b) forms a horizontal axis in the body
   c) is composed of the skull, ribs, and vertebra
   d) is the major division containing the largest number of bones

2. Which of the following cranial bones does not form the calvaria?
   a) parietal
   b) temporal
   c) ethmoid
   d) frontal

3. Which of the following facial bones does not form a part of the nasal cavity?
   a) ethmoid
   b) zygomatic
   c) vomer
   d) inferior conchae

4. Which of the following is not a bone forming the orbit?
   a) lacrimal
   b) sphenoid
   c) ethmoid
   d) occipital

5. A foramen, process, tubercle, and facet are all examples of:
   a) articulations
   b) surface features
   c) joints
   d) All of the above

6. Most of the facial bones, and the arm and leg bones, are classified on the basis of their embryological development as:
   a) alveolar
   b) dermal
   c) cancellous
   d) endoskeletal

7. Which of the following is true of a long bone?
   a) the shaft or main body is called the epiphysis
   b) each end terminates in a region called the diaphysis
   c) the diaphysis grows in opposite directions to elongate the bone
   d) All of the above

8. Bone matrix is composed of:
   a) osteocalcin
   b) hydroxylapatite
   c) collagen fiber
   d) All of the above

9. Compact, or cortical, bone
   a) makes up about 80% of the bones in the human body.
   b) is composed of microscopic structural units called osteons.
   c) contributes only a small proportion of bone weight.
   d) forms the ends of long bones and the center of other bones.

10. Which of the following best describes synovial fluid?
    a) is found in bursa
    b) lubricates joint linings
    c) is found in synovial capsules
    d) All of the above

11. Which of the following is the correct order in the process of endochondrial bone formation?
    a) bone collar formation, cartilage peg formation, epiphysial osteoclast activity
    b) cartilage peg formation, bone collar formation, epiphsial osteoclast activity
    c) epiphysial osteoclast activity, bone collar formation, secondary ossification
    d) osteoclast activity at cartilage pegs, secondary ossification, bone collar formation

12. The five stages of endochondrial bone formation can be "condensed" to three phases known as:
    a) reactive, reparative, and restorative
    b) initiating, rebuilding, and molding
    c) reaction, repair, and shaping
    d) response, resourcing, and restoration

13. Which of the following best describes shin splints?
    a) are a type of stress fracture
    b) involve the bone tissue of the tibia
    c) result from abnormal stretching of the ligaments and tendons
    d) All of the above

14. Tooth decay includes:
    a) loss of calcium from teeth
    b) formation of cavities
    c) loss of collagen connective tissue
    d) All of the above

15. Myeloma is cancer of:
    a) red blood cells
    b) red bone marrow
    c) bone cells
    d) white blood cells

16. Which of the following skeletal system conditions is due to loss of blood flow?
    a) osteonecrosis
    b) scleroderma
    c) osteomyelitis
    d) osteomalacia

17. Match the letter of each type of joint with the best description of the movement it allows:

    a) amphiarthrosis   _____ widest variety of movements

    b) diarthrosis   _____ only slight movement

    c) synarthrosis   _____ no movement

18. Match the letter of each type of synarthrosis with the best clue pertaining to it:

    a) gomphosis   _____ ligaments

    b) synchondrosis   _____ bone fusion

    c) syndesmosis   _____ cartilage

    d) synostosis   _____ socket

19. Match the letter of each type of bone fracture with the clue that pertains to it:

    a) comminuted (compound)   _____ skin tearing

    b) greenstick   _____ bone displacement

    c) open   _____ very small

    d) simple   _____ break and bend of bone

    e) stress   _____ cracked bone only

20. Match the letter of each type of arthritis with the clue that pertains to it.

    a) ankylosing spondylitis   _____ affects cartilage at bone ends

    b) rheumatoid arthritis   _____ affects spine articular cartilage

    c) osteoarthritis   _____ autoimmune attack of connective tissue

21. For each bone shape, list the type of ossification that usually occurs during its development:

    long bones:

    flat bones:

    irregular:

22. List five categories of synovial joints (based on the motion permitted by each), and name two bones that are articulated by each type.

a)

b)

c)

d)

e)

23. Place the following stages of bone healing in the proper order of occurrence during bone repair in the body: callus, granulation, lamellar bone, fracture, and normal contour.

24. List three factors that are thought to contribute to osteoporosis.

25. List four factors that can contribute to aging of the skeletal system.

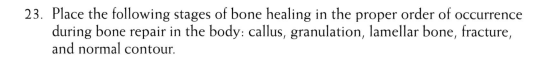

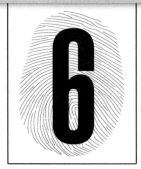

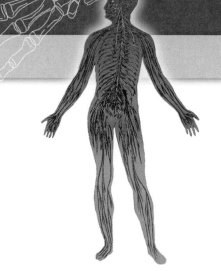

CHAPTER

6

THE MUSCULAR SYSTEM

Completion

Complete the following sentences by filling in each blank with a key term from the text.

1. Muscle cells can be classified three ways: 1) _____, 2) type of _____, and 3) _____.

2. The contractile unit of a muscle cell is called a _____, which is composed of an overlapping pattern of thick and thin _____.

3. Skeletal muscle contraction is initiated by the nerve cell release of the neurotransmitter _____, which binds to a _____ on the muscle cell's membrane or _____.

4. A resting muscle cell normally has a higher intracellular ion concentration of _____ and a higher extracellular concentration of _____. These levels are maintained by a system called the _____ _____.

5. Skeletal muscle contraction occurs in three stages: 1) _____, 2) _____, and 3) _____.

6. The immovable muscle attachment point is called the _____, and the connection to the body part that moves during a muscle contraction is called the _____.

7. The three levels of muscle structure are 1) _____, 2) _____, and 3) _____.

8. _____ describes a muscle action of active lengthening or shortening while _____ describes action with no change in muscle length.

59

9. _____ muscle fibers are referred to as white because they contain only small amounts of _____. They are referred to metabolically as _____ because they undergo _____ respiration.

10. _____ muscle fibers are referred to as red because they contain large amounts of _____. They are referred to metabolically as _____ because they undergo _____ respiration.

Matching

Match each of the following terms with the clue that best describes it by placing the letter of the term in the blank next to the correct clue.

a) antagonistic

b) cachexia

c) cardiac muscle

d) contractile proteins

e) creatine phosphate

f) fascicle

g) motor

h) myoglobin

i) neuromuscular junction

j) nonstriated

k) sarcolemma

l) smooth muscle

m) sphincter

n) sprain

o) Type 2b fibers

_____ random pattern of contractile proteins

_____ found in digestive organs and blood vessels

_____ nerves that control skeletal muscle

_____ intrinsic beat

_____ muscle cell membrane

_____ space between a nerve cell and sarcolemma

_____ stores energy in muscle cells

_____ a bundle of muscle fibers

_____ muscle action that resists another muscle

_____ decrease in the size of an opening

_____ fast glycolytic

_____ type of muscle injury

_____ muscle loss

_____ stores oxygen for aerobic respiration of muscle

_____ causes muscle cell cytoskeleton to contract

Complete the Terms Table

Complete the missing key terms and/or definitions in the following table.

Term	Definition
	embryological development of muscle tissue from mesoderm cells
myofilaments	
myofibrils	
	system of the inner membrane of muscle cells that stores and transports calcium for muscle contraction
rigor mortis	
	the stable, immovable point of attachment of a muscle
	connective tissue covering gross muscle
synergistic	
rotator	
	muscle fiber type also known as slow oxidative due to its metabolic activity of aerobic respiration
	abnormal involuntary muscle movement
cramp	
myopathy	
	calcium imbalance disease that causes arm and leg spasms
muscular dystrophies	

Label the Graphic

Identify each of the following terms in the illustration on page 62. Write the number of the anatomical part on the line pointing to its location.

1. biceps brachii (arm)
2. biceps femoris (thigh)
3. deltoid
4. frontal
5. gastrocnemius
6. gluteal muscles
7. gracilis
8. infraspinous
9. latissimus dorsi
10. occipital
11. orbicularis oculi (eye)
12. orbicularis oris (mouth)
13. pectoral
14. quadriceps
15. rectus abdominis
16. sartorius
17. semimembranous
18. semitendinosus
19. splenius
20. sternocleidomastoid
21. temporal
22. teres muscles
23. tibialis anterior
24. trapezius
25. triceps brachii

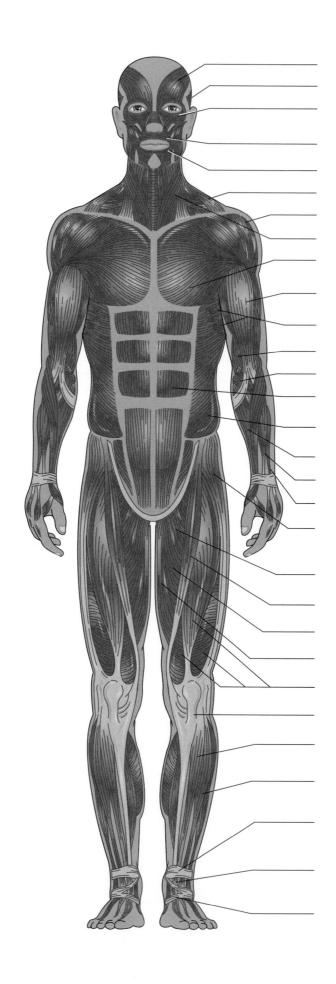

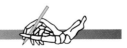

Color the Graphic

Color this illustration using the following color key:

muscle – pink
tendon – brown
fasciculi – red
muscle fiber – orange
single myofibril – purple

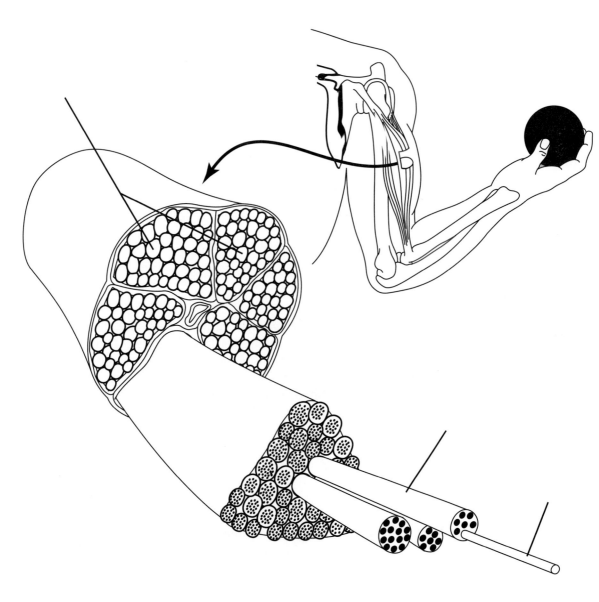

63

Practical Application

Write brief responses to the following scenarios.

1. How would stimulation of smooth muscle contraction affect blood pressure, air inhalation, and defecation (i.e., evacuation of food waste from the digestive tract)?

2. Sympathetic nerve activity is usually associated with the phrase "flight or fight." This often leads to the misconception that it is only excitatory in nature. What would be inaccurate about this assumption?

3. An enzyme called acetylcholinesterase enzymatically breaks down acetylcholine at the neuromuscular synapse. Would an anticholinesterase drug (an inhibitor of this enzyme) cause an increase or decrease in skeletal muscle activity? Would this effect be described as blocking or increasing sympathetic nerve activity?

4. What are the two major antagonistic muscle groups located proximally on the lower appendages? (Use Figure 6.10a and Figure 6.10b as a reference.) Given their locations and actions, which attachment points do you think they might have in common, and describe why the contraction of each muscle results in the described action (include the terms *origin* and *insertion* in your answer).

5. Why is skeletal muscle multinucleated?

6. When the diaphragm muscle contracts, its position in the body is lowered. In contrast, when the external intercostal muscles of the ribs contract, they become elevated. Both of these muscle contractions create more volume in the thoracic cavity. The resultant decrease in the pressure within the thoracic cavity causes air to move from the body's exterior (where there is higher pressure) into the lower-pressure area of the thoracic cavity. Thus, inspiration occurs as the lungs fill with air. Relaxing of these muscle returns them to their original positions, and exhaling forces air out. Given this information about the mechanics of inspiration, how might the calcium leakage into the sarcomeres (as occurs following death) of diaphragm muscle tissue explain the phenomenom of a corpse making a "moaning" sound?

7. The deltoid muscle "caps" the shoulder. Its origin is on the bones of the shoulder girdle, and its insertion is on the deltoid tuberosity which is located on the lateral side of the humerus. On the basis of this information, provide the term of muscle movement that would describe its action and explain how this occurs. What muscle movement term would describe the action of muscles antagonistic to the deltoid?

8. Would the muscles that cause flexion of the neck have their origin or their insertion on the head? Explain your reasoning.

9. Classify each of the following activities as either isometric or isotonic, and briefly explain your answers: 1) biceps curls; and 2) balancing on tip toes.

10. Relate the condition of myolitis ossificans to the meaning of each of the "subparts."

Crossword Puzzle

Complete the following crossword puzzle using key terms from the text.

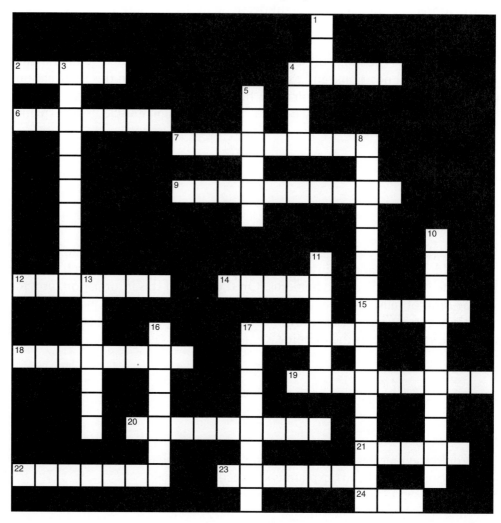

Across

2. anchors the sarcomere to the sarcolemma
4. muscle cells
6. smaller muscle group
7. movable muscle attachment point
9. connective tissue of muscle fascicles
12. triangular muscle shape
14. color of Type 2b muscle fibers
15. thin myofibril protein
17. thick myofibril protein
18. source of glucose for muscles
19. reduces sex hormone production
20. Type 2b muscle fiber respiration
21. located between myosin and actin filaments
22. longest of a muscle group
23. "feather-patterned" muscle
24. color of Type 1 muscle fibers

Down

1. indirect measure of body density
3. cell membrane protein that allows permeability to ions
4. speed of Type 2a muscle fibers
5. shortest of a muscle group
8. nerve cell chemical for cell communication
10. moves food through the digestive tract
11. causes a body part to be more rigid
13. has three origins
16. rigid-paralysis disease
17. abnormally slow muscle relaxation

Quiz

1. Striations are produced by the uniform arrangement of:

   a) muscle fibers
   b) sarcomeres
   c) fascicles
   d) All of the above

2. What percentage of the body's mass is composed of muscle tissue?

   a) 25
   b) 10
   c) 75
   d) 50

3. Muscles can be categorized as:

   a) striated and nonstriated
   b) involuntary and voluntary
   c) cardiac, skeletal, and smooth
   d) All of the above

4. When a muscle cell is contracted, microscopic observation would reveal:

   a) overlap of thick and thin filaments
   b) increased distance between the Z lines
   c) lack of striations
   d) All of the above

5. The three proteins in thin myofilaments are:

   a) myosin, titin, and actin
   b) tropomyosin, troponin, and myosin
   c) actin, tropomyosin, and troponin
   d) titin, myosin, and tropomyosin

6. Cell-muscle contraction is initiated by nerve cell release of:

   a) epinephrine
   b) troponin
   c) calcium
   d) acetylcholine

7. The muscle cell contraction phase begins when the sarcoplasmic reticulum releases _____, which binds to the protein _____ on the thin myofilaments.

   a) acetylcholine/receptors
   b) calcium/troponin
   c) potassium/myosin
   d) sodium/ion channels

8. During muscle cell relaxation there is:

   a) no continued neural stimulation of the sarcolemma
   b) calcium release
   c) special neurotransmitter release for muscle lengthening
   d) All of the above

9. The Z line of the sarcomere:

   a) connects the thick and thin filaments
   b) anchors the sarcomeres to the sarcolemma
   c) forms the sarcoplasmic reticulum
   d) All of the above

10. Which of the following orders is correct in placing the terms of muscle anatomy in order from the smallest to the largest?

    a) myofilament, myofibril, muscle fiber, and fascicle
    b) myofibril, myofilament, fascicle, and muscle fiber
    c) fascicle, myofilament, myofibril, and muscle fiber
    d) muscle fiber, fascicle, myofibril, and myofilament

11. Which of the following is involved in energy storage for muscle contraction?

    a) creatine phosphate
    b) glycogen
    c) myoglobin
    d) All of the above

12. When a muscle contracts, the insertion:

    a) remains stationary
    b) moves toward the origin
    c) detaches
    d) has no functional role

13. Type 2b fibers:

    a) fatigue easily
    b) undergo anaerobic respiration
    c) create lactic acid
    d) All of the above

14. Isotonic muscle action involves:

    a) only muscles of the appendages
    b) active lengthening and shortening
    c) isolation of muscle fibers
    d) All of the above

15. Type 1 fibers:

    a) undergo aerobic respiration
    b) are white
    c) have small amounts of myoglobin
    d) All of the above

16. Which answer best describes Type 2a fibers?

    a) are slow oxidative
    b) are white
    c) undergo both aerobic and anaerobic respiration
    d) All of the above

17. Mitochondrial myopathies prevent muscle cells from producing:

    a) glucose
    b) oxygen
    c) energy
    d) creatine phosphate

18. Muscular dystrophies:

    a) result in muscle atrophy
    b) usually result from inadequate innervation
    c) are characterized by progressive muscle wasting
    d) All of the above

19. Match the letter of each of the gross-muscle shapes to the description that best fits.

    a) rhomboideus _____ saw toothed
    b) serratus _____ diamond shaped
    c) trapezius _____ triangular

20. Match each of the following types of muscle action with the description that best describes it.

    a) abductor _____ produces a downward movement
    b) depressor _____ turns the palm downward
    c) flexor _____ decreases the angle of a joint
    d) pronator _____ moves a body part away from the midline

21. Match each of the following types of muscle action with its antagonist.

    a) abductor _____ levator
    b) depressor _____ supinator
    c) flexor _____ adductor
    d) pronator _____ extensor

22. List three aging factors that contribute to cachexia.

23. List the three types of muscle connective tissue along with the structure that they cover.

24. List the three types of muscle tissue classified by their location in the body.

25. Differentiate between rigid and flaccid paralysis.

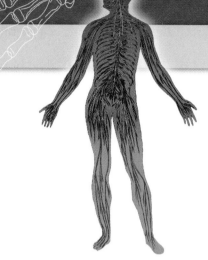

7 ENDOCRINE GLANDS AND HORMONES

Completion

Complete the following sentences by filling in each blank with a key term from the text.

1. Secretions that circulate to their target organ are produced by _____ glands while secretions that enter a body area through a duct are produced by _____ glands.

2. Some hormones reach _____ receptors via transport by carrier proteins.

3. Most _____ hormones attach to external receptors, but _____ hormones dissolve across the cell membrane and bind to receptors inside the cell.

4. Nerve cells of the hypothalamus produce chemicals called _____, which travel to the _____ _____ gland to stimulate its production of hormones.

5. _____ decreases blood calcium levels while _____ _____ increases blood calcium levels.

6. _____ cells of the pancreas produce _____, which _____ blood glucose levels, while _____ cells of the pancreas produce _____, which _____ blood glucose levels.

7. The pineal gland produces both _____, a hormone involved in digestion, emotion, and sleep, and _____, a hormone stimulated by sunlight which regulates body rhythms.

8. The cortex of the adrenal gland produces two major groups of hormones called _____ and _____, while the adrenal medulla produces _____ and _____.

71

9. An abnormally low level of adrenal cortex hormone production can result in the disease _____, while overproduction of these hormones is the cause of _____.

10. The hormone most commonly involved in hormone replacement therapy is _____; its presence in _____ makes this food a natural alternative sought by many to counteract diminished production of the hormone during the _____ process.

Matching

Match each of the following terms with the clue that best describes it by placing the letter of the term in the blank next to the correct clue.

a) aldosterone   _____ produces antidiuretic hormone

b) antagonist   _____ stimulates uterine contractions

c) autocrine   _____ produces thyroxin

d) cortisol   _____ secretion that allows cellular self-control

e) diabetes insipidus   _____ insufficient thyroxine production

f) follicle-stimulating hormone   _____ detect specific hormone secretion

g) Graves' disease   _____ controls lipid and protein metabolism

h) hypothyroidism   _____ allow cells to detect stimuli

i) oxytocin   _____ regulates potassium and sodium levels

j) posterior pituitary   _____ blocks hormone action

k) progesterone   _____ promotes the formation of eggs and sperm

l) receptors   _____ insufficient antidiuretic hormone production

m) target cells   _____ inflammation of the thyroid

n) thymus   _____ menstrual cycle regulation and pregnancy

o) thyroid   _____ stimulates T-cell production

Complete the Terms Table

Complete the missing key terms and/or definitions in the following table.

Term	Definition
	embryological development of muscle tissue from mesoderm cells
	the interior region of the adrenal glands
	hormone produced by the anterior pituitary that stimulates the adrenal cortex
agonist	
antidiuretic hormone	
	disease caused by either insufficient insulin production or faulty insulin receptors
growth hormone	
	chemical secretion produced inside the body that acts as a stimulus to initiate a response
islets	
ligand	
	secretions that travel via the blood or body fluids to their target cells
	endocrine gland that is responsible for increasing blood calcium levels
pheromones	
	hormone secreted by the kidneys in response to a decrease in blood pressure
	hormone produced by the thymus gland that stimulates T-cell differentiation in white blood cells
thyroxine	

Label the Graphic

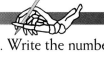

Identify each of the following terms in the illustration on page 74. Write the number of the anatomical part on the line pointing to its location.

1. anterior pituitary
2. posterior pituitary
3. nerve connection to the hypothalamus

Place the number for each of the following terms of the pituitary gland hormones in the correct space to indicate its respective target organ.

4. adrenocorticotropic hormone
5. antidiuretic hormone
6. follicle-stimulating hormone
7. growth hormone
8. luteinizing hormone
9. melanocyte-stimulating hormone
10. oxytocin
11. prolactin
12. thyroid-stimulating hormone

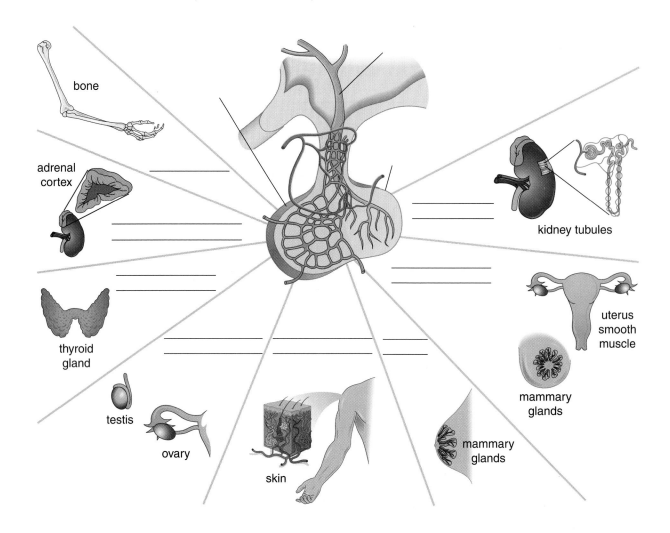

bone

adrenal
cortex

thyroid
gland

testis

ovary

skin

kidney tubules

uterus
smooth
muscle

mammary
glands

mammary
glands

1. Are all endocrine organs under the control of the pituitary gland? Why or why not?

2. Are all hormones in the body produced by endocrine system organs? Explain.

Color the Graphic

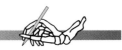

Color this illustration using the following color key:

adrenal – red
hypothalamus – pink
pancreas – yellow
parathyroid – black
pineal – dark green
pituitary – purple
thymus – light blue
thyroid – orange
ovaries – light green
testes – brown

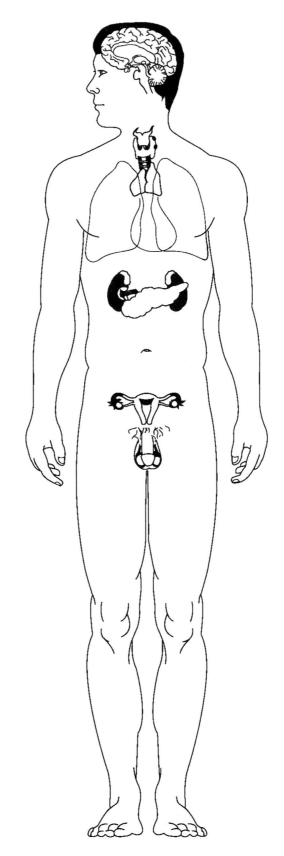

75

Practical Application

Write brief responses to the following scenarios.

1. The pituitary gland is known as the master gland. What is the reason for this description, and is it truly the "control" center for the majority for endocrine system hormone production?

2. What does the neural innervation of the hypothalamus (Figure 7.9) indicate about the effect is has on the pituitary? Address the description of the pituitary as a "double organ" in your answer.

3. Notice the arrangement of the capillary system that leads to the pituitary gland (Figure 7.9). Does this arrangement indicate anything about the control the hypothalamus has over the pituitary gland?

4. Why could a disease that affects the pituitary gland have a negative effect on the adrenal gland?

5. Explain why a particular hormone exerts its effects only on certain cells. In addition, describe how the endocrine system can be "fooled" at the receptor level.

6. Give two different roles that the cardiovascular system plays in the proper functioning of the endocrine system.

7. The use of a hand and wrist x-ray of a child might be beneficial in the detection of which hormone deficiency?

8. In addition to the symptoms of Addison's disease described in the text, another peculiar symptom of this disease is a tanned appearance of the skin. (Interestingly, President John F. Kennedy had this disease which, ironically, explains his "healthy" suntanned look.) Elevation of adrenocorticotropic hormone (ACTH) is the source of this symptom. In high levels this hormone actually stimulates the receptors of another anterior pituitary hormone that causes the darkening of skin. Explain why ACTH would be elevated in this disease, and name the anterior pituitary hormone with which it "competes" to cause the darkened skin appearance.

9. Urine tests can aid in identifying certain pathologies. A common urine analysis test can be used to detect glucose in the urine, which is an indicator of diabetes mellitus. (In persons with diabetes, normal blood glucose levels are metabolized at a rate that prevents them from being excreted.) Why would a person with this disease be excreting glucose? What else might be detected in elevated levels in the urine?

10. The normal level of which mineral would be affected by hypoparathyroidism? Would you expect this mineral to become deficient or excessive in the body, and what other body systems would be most adversely affected?

Crossword Puzzle

Complete the following crossword puzzle using key terms from the text.

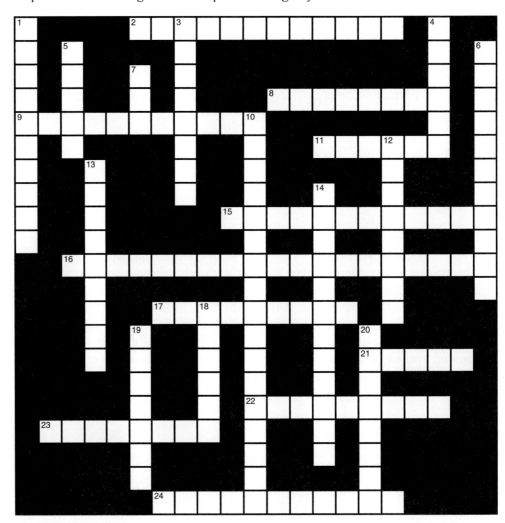

Across

2. the part of the brain that controls the pituitary
8. primary glucocorticosteroid
9. located on the thyroid gland
11. the sex organs
15. hormone produced by the testes
16. examples are sunlight, temperature, and nutrients
17. the master gland
21. hormone type that dissolves across cell membranes
22. stimulates milk production
23. these glands' secretions travel through blood
24. regulates sodium and potassium levels

Down

1. another name for the pituitary gland
3. produces insulin and glucagon
4. white blood cells associated with thymosin
5. produces estrogen and progesterone
6. sites of hormone-receptor binding
7. short for the hormone that stimulates egg and sperm production
10. caused by inadequate ADH levels
12. part of pituitary that produces ACTH, GH, LH, FSH, TSH, MSH, and pro-lactin
13. epinephrine
14. norepinephrine
18. endocrine organ located above the heart
19. lowers blood glucose levels
20. raises blood glucose levels

1. _____ True or False: All glands of the endocrine system function exclusively for hormone production.

2. The number of endocrine glands (consider a "paired" gland as one) composing the endocrine system is:

   a) twelve
   b) eight
   c) six
   d) nine

3. Endocrine glands produce secretions:

   a) that travel directly to the body area they affect
   b) used only by other endocrine glands
   c) in response to signals from the environment or from other cells
   d) All of the above

4. Hormones produced by endocrine glands reach their target cells because:

   a) target cells have specialized receptors that detect specific hormones
   b) specialized capillary systems direct specific hormones to specific locations
   c) hormones can be sent directly through ducts connecting endocrine organs to their target cells
   d) All of the above

5. Which of the following statements could be considered to be true?

   a) When a hormone binds to a receptor it causes biochemical changes to the target cell.
   b) Hormones are stimuli that when detected by receptors elicit a response from an effector.
   c) Target cells possess receptors and act as effectors.
   d) All of the above

6. Hormone receptors categorized as internal when they:

   a) interact with a specific portion of the carrier proteins DNA when stimulated
   b) rely on carrier proteins to receive their specific hormones
   c) are located on the cell membrane
   d) All of the above

7. Endocrine system secretions described as autocrine:

   a) regulate other endocrine organs
   b) leave the body and signal cells of other organisms
   c) do not travel through the blood to reach their target cells
   d) travel via body fluids to their receptor cells

8. The negative feedback system that many endocrine glands utilize:

   a) is a type of self-regulation
   b) ensures that hormone production will continue until "shut-off" by another body system
   c) relies on exocrine-gland interaction
   d) All of the above

9. Chemicals that can act as hormones:

   a) may be medically advantageous
   b) may be considered environmental risk factors
   c) are sometimes referred to as hormone mimics
   d) All of the above

10. Insufficient levels of cholesterol in the body might interfere with the production of:

    a) any peptide hormone
    b) steroids
    c) all lipid hormones
    d) All of the above

11. Which of the following statements is true?

    a) lipid hormones and peptide hormones play equal roles in long-term body effects
    b) most lipid hormones usually have a short-term influence on the body
    c) most lipid hormones have long-term effects on the body
    d) protein hormones cannot be removed from the body

12. The pituitary gland:

    a) is self-regulated
    b) is under control of the hypothalamus
    c) is stimulated by hormones of other endocrine glands
    d) All of the above

13. The posterior pituitary gland produces:

    a) hormones that influence water loss
    b) hormones that influence many other endocrine organs
    c) hormones involved in self-regulation
    d) All of the above

14. Leutinizing hormone stimulates:

    a) gamete production in both sexes
    b) sperm production only
    c) egg production only
    d) production of estrogen and testosterone

15. Which of the following would most likely occur from abnormal growth hormone production?

    a) no serious results, due to compensation by other endocrine glands
    b) dwarfism or gigantism
    c) effects on reproductive capabilities only
    d) atrophy of the pituitary gland

16. Light therapy can be used to treat symptoms that result from lack of :

   a) prolactin
   b) ACTH
   c) melatonin
   d) ADH

17. Glucocorticoids and minerocorticoids are produced by the:

   a) kidneys
   b) anterior pituitary
   c) adrenal medulla
   d) adrenal cortex

18. The production of epinephrine and norepinephrine:

   a) occurs in the adrenal medulla
   b) is initiated in response to stress, heavy physical exertion, or low blood glucose
   c) initiates release of glucose and fat into the blood
   d) All of the above

19. Low levels of thyroxine production would most likely result in:

   a) weight gain
   b) elevated body temperatures
   c) increased heart rate
   d) All of the above

20. Blood calcium levels are controlled by:

   a) the thyroid gland
   b) the parathyroid glands
   c) calcitonin
   d) All of the above

21. Damage to the beta cells of the pancreas would most likely result in:

   a) decreased insulin production
   b) decreased glucagon production
   c) decreased blood glucose levels
   d) All of the above

22. Abnormal T-cell production would indicate abnormality of which endocrine organ?

   a) the thyroid
   b) the parathyroids
   c) the thymus
   d) All of the above

23. Which of the following diseases can be thought of as opposites?

   a) diabetes mellitus and diabetes insipidus
   b) Cushing's disease and Addison's disease
   c) Grave's disease and hyperthyroidism
   d) hypoactive growth-hormone production and dwarfism

ENDOCRINE GLANDS AND HORMONES

24. The sex hormones:

    a) are elevated during puberty
    b) exert influence during fetal development
    c) are decreased in older age
    d) All of the above

25. Aging of the digestive system effects endocrine function because:

    a) digestion requires increased energy
    b) elevated hormones are excreted from the body
    c) absorption of certain nutrients necessary for hormone production is decreased
    d) neural innervation necessary for hormone activity is lost

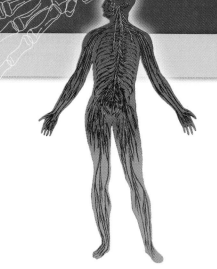

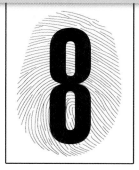

8 FUNCTION OF THE NERVOUS SYSTEM

Completion

Complete the following sentences by filling in each blank with a key term from the text.

1. _____ are categorized by their cell anatomy, while _____ are classified by the way in which they assist nerve cells.

2. Four common features of all neurons are: the _____, _____, _____, and _____.

3. _____ can only receive information from other cells, while _____ transmit information but can also receive information through an _____.

4. Most _____ neurons produce only one type of neurotransmitter, but _____ neurons can contain a variety of neurotransmitter receptors.

5. Neurons are described as one of three primary shapes: _____, _____, and _____.

6. Neuroglia called astrocytes help form a protective feature called the _____, while ependymal-cell neuroglia produce _____.

7. The _____ charge inside the cell is -70 millivolts (mV), but when an _____ occurs, the increased flow of sodium into the cell causes the cell to reach a stage called _____.

8. _____ neurotransmitters cause the sodium channels to open, which initiates an action potential, while _____ neurotransmitters make it more difficult for the neuron to achieve an action potential.

9. In a reflex arc the _____ receives stimuli, while the _____ responds to it.

10. Nerve cell diseases can be categorized into five major groups: infectious, degenerative, _____, _____, and _____.

Matching

Match each of the following terms with the clue that best describes it by placing the letter of the term in the blank next to the correct clue.

a) amyotropical lateral sclerosis (ALS)

b) catecholamine

c) cytokines

d) gamma amniobutiric acid (GABA)

e) hyperpolarization

f) internal stimuli

g) interneurons

h) lipofuscin

i) neurotrophic

j) propagate

k) Schwann cells

l) soma

m) synaptic cleft

n) threshold

o) terminus

_____ produce myelin

_____ to travel across

_____ cell secretions used to communicate information

_____ point of sodium-channel opening

_____ excitatory neurotransmitter

_____ gap at the nerve terminus

_____ inhibitory amino acid neurotransmitter

_____ indicates nerve cell pathology

_____ nerve cell body

_____ bipolar neuron dendrites

_____ genetic degenerative disorder

_____ maintain cell health and activity

_____ more negative potential than resting potential

_____ capable of invading neurons

_____ site of neurotransmitter release

Complete the Terms Table

Complete the missing key terms and/or definitions in the following table.

Term	Definition
	environmental factors that influence metabolic changes in a cell or physiological changes in tissues and organs
neural tube	
	region of the nerve cell body from which the axon extends
	neuron cell extensions that receive stimuli
	neuroglial cells that help maintain the chemical environment of neurons and may help in nerve cell repair
nodes of Ranvier	

	the action potential stage following repolarization during which a normal stimulation will not cause another action potential
tetany	
	catecholamine neurotransmitter that can be inhibitory as well as excitatory
innervate	
reverberating pathway	
	involuntary responses to a stimulus
	inflammation of membranes surrounding the brain
	a neurotrophic disease caused by infectious prions that can be contracted through exposure to the blood and meat of infected animals
tonic control	

Label the Graphic

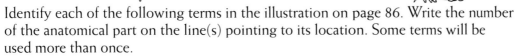

Identify each of the following terms in the illustration on page 86. Write the number of the anatomical part on the line(s) pointing to its location. Some terms will be used more than once.

1. axon
2. cell body
3. collaterals
4. dendrite(s)
5. muscle fiber
6. myelin sheath
7. nodes of Ranvier

1. How would you describe each of the illustrated neuron types (motor, interneuron, sensory) by shape (i.e., unipolar, bipolar, or multipolar)?

2. In what order would the neuron types be arranged in a reflex arc?

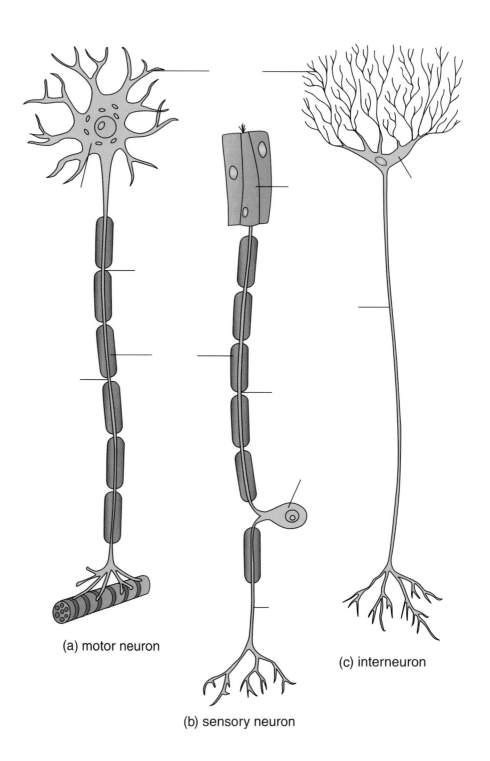

(a) motor neuron

(b) sensory neuron

(c) interneuron

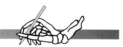

Color the Graphic

Color this illustration using the following color key:

Neuroglial cells

    astrocytes – red

    ependymal cells – pink

    microglial cells – yellow

    oligodendrites – green

Neuron anatomy

    axons – light blue

    dendrites – brown

    myelin sheath – dark blue

    soma – orange

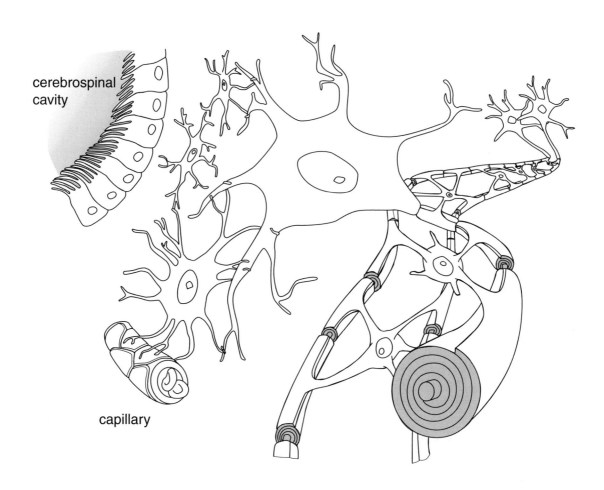

cerebrospinal cavity

capillary

1. Does this illustration represent nervous tissue in the central nervous system or in the peripheral nervous system? Give the evidence for your answer.

FUNCTION OF THE NERVOUS SYSTEM

Practical Application

Write brief responses to the following scenarios.

1. Describe a typical reflex arc in terms of the most likely shape of each neuron at each of the three "portions" of the arc.

2. How can the same neurotransmitter be described as being both excitatory and inhibitory?

3. Can a chemical synapse cause an action potential to occur in both directions of a neural pathway?

4. Describe the action potential terms depolarize, hyperpolarize, and repolarize relative to resting potential. For each indicate what change has occurred to cause the membrane potential measurement of each.

5. Would a drug described as antagonistic to a neurotransmitter increase or decrease the normal neurotransmitter response? What might be the mechanism of such a drug if it were to exert its effects on the postsynaptic side of the synaptic cleft?

6. What type of pathology might be indicated by the presence of an extremely high number of microglial cells in the nervous system?

7. Compare and contrast Schwann cells and oligodendritic cells.

8. Epilepsy is characterized by uncontrolled excitatory neuronal activity. Could this disease be caused by a lack of glutamate or of GABA?

9. The disease amyotrophic lateral sclerosis (ALS) is characterized by scar tissue that forms sclerotic (hardened) areas in the spinal cord that control the diaphragm and intercostal muscles. This damage results in a progressive loss of innervation to these muscles. Why would this disease be fatal?

10. Neurons are more susceptible to the negative consequences of aging than are many other types of cells in the body. Briefly discuss two characteristics of neuron cells that contribute to this vulnerability.

Crossword Puzzle

Complete the following crossword puzzle using key terms from the text.

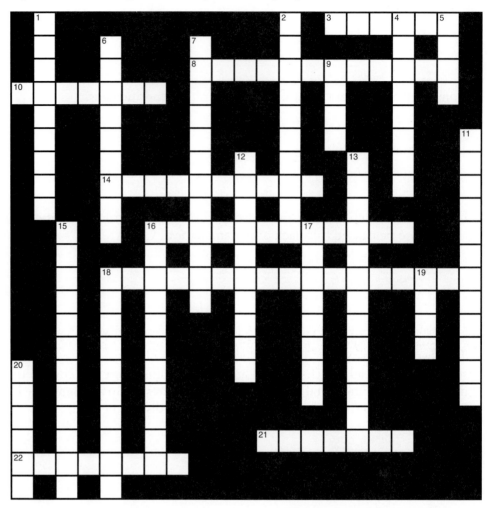

Across

3. disease caused by lack of galactosylce-ramide beta-galactosidase
8. brain inflammation
10. accumlated materials in cells
14. describes synapse between the termi-nus and a nerve cell body
16. acetylcholine is an example of this neurotransmitter type
18. disease resulting from loss of Schwann cells
21. altered nerve cell cytoplasm
22. disease of uncontrolled excitatory neu-ral activity

Down

1. autonomic nerve response pathway
2. return to resting potential
4. bacterial disease causing flaccid paralysis
5. Abbr: action potential of postsynaptic neuron caused by this

6. excitatory amino acid neurotransmit-ter
7. neuron poison found in frogs and puffer fish
9. transmits stimuli to the terminus
11. disease caused by lack of intestinal nerve cells
12. organize neuron interconnections
13. communication between neurons and neuroglia
15. describes synapse between the termi-nus and a "receiving" cell extension
16. axon branches
17. follows refractory period
18. serotonin and histamine are examples of this type of neurotransmitter
19. nerve cell body
20. viral neural disease transmitted through infected animal saliva

Quiz

1. _____ True or False: Neuroglial cells are the only cells of the nervous system thought to function in nerve cell repair.

2. Sunlight would be an example of:

    a) an affector
    b) an external stimulus
    c) a receptor
    d) All of the above

3. Which of the following best describes neurons and neuroglia?

    a) function independently of one another
    b) are distributed in equal numbers throughout the nervous system
    c) are derived from neural stem cells
    d) All of the above

4. The synaptic cleft could be located at:

    a) a dendrite of a presynaptic neuron
    b) the terminus of a postsynaptic neuron
    c) the terminus of a presynaptic neuron
    d) All of the above

5. Motor neurons are:

    a) unipolar
    b) multipolar
    c) bipolar
    d) All of the above

6. Which of the following neuroglial types could be described as the "gatekeeper" between the vascular and nervous systems?

    a) Schwann cells
    b) satellite cells
    c) astrocytes
    d) ependymal cells

7. Which of the following best describes a cell at resting potential?

    a) is more positively charged inside than is its surrounding environment
    b) is more negatively charged inside than is its surrounding environment
    c) has a charge equivalent to its external environment
    d) is not in an excitable condition

8. At threshold, the cytoplasm's charge is :

    a) more negative than at resting potential
    b) becoming more negative due to gaining potassium
    c) changing due to loss of sodium
    d) more positive than at resting potential

9. Depolarization:

    a) is characterized by the cell's interior being more positive than the exterior
    b) precedes repolarization
    c) accompanies the release of the neurotransmitter into the synaptic cleft
    d) All of the above

10. Action potential propagation is sped up by:

    a) the influx of calcium
    b) the presence of myelin sheaths along the axon
    c) hyperpolarization
    d) All of the above

11. Which of the following best describes neurotransmitters?

    a) are released by the presynaptic neuron
    b) transfer the action potential from a sensory neuron to a motor neuron
    c) can be excitatory or inhibitory
    d) All of the above

12. Neurotransmitters that are similar to the hormones made by the adrenal medulla are classified as:

    a) monoamines
    b) catecholamines
    c) amino-acid derivatives
    d) cholinergic

13. A diet void of fat would decrease the production of which of the following neurotransmitters?

    a) serotonin
    b) dopamine
    c) acetylcholine
    d) All of the above

14. Which of the following best describes a reverberating neural pathway?

    a) It is a type of axon self-stimulation.
    b) It is inhibitory.
    c) It results from an axosomatic synapse.
    d) All of the above

15. Reflexes:

    a) are involuntary neural responses
    b) are controlled by a neural pathway called a reflex arc
    c) transmit stimuli from the environment through an afferent neuron
    d) All of the above

16. Interneurons of a reflex arc are responsible for:

    a) detecting the initial stimulus
    b) consciously modifying certain reflexes
    c) directly innervating a muscle or gland
    d) All of the above

17. Flaccid paralysis might result from:

    a) excessive production of excitatory neurotransmitter
    b) excessive production of catecholamine
    c) loss of acetylcholine reuptake
    d) inability of acetylcholine to bind to postsynaptic receptors

18. Which of the following would most likely result from the production of bacterial endotoxin?

    a) inflammation
    b) paralysis
    c) demyelination
    d) All of the above

19. Which of the following diseases would be acquired before birth? :

    a) Krabbe's disease
    b) Lou Gehrig's disease (ALS)
    c) Hirschsprung's disease
    d) All of the above

20. Creutzfeldt-Jakob disease is:

    a) caused by prions
    b) similar to mad cow disease
    c) transmissible through contact with certain body tissues
    d) All of the above

21. Herpes can be categorized as a disease that is:

    a) neurotrophic
    b) infectious
    c) degenerative
    d) All of the above

22. Certain types of infectious disease could also be classified as:

    a) toxicological
    b) traumatic
    c) developmental
    d) All of the above

23. Traumatic injury resulting in neuron loss can be repaired by:

    a) damaged neurons undergoing mitosis
    b) associated neuroglial cells
    c) macrophages
    d) All of the above

24. Which of the following statements is true?

    a) Neuron cells replicate throughout an individual's life.
    b) Neuron cells have a relatively low metabolic rate.
    c) The number of neurons an individual has does not change throughout their life span.
    d) When a neuron dies it cannot be replaced.

25. Which of the following is a result of nerve cell aging?

a) loss of tonic control
b) decreased blood flow
c) oxidation by metabolic waste products
d) decreased nutrient absorption

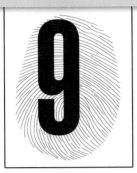

STRUCTURE OF THE NERVOUS SYSTEM

Completion

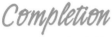

Complete the following sentences by filling in each blank with a key term from the text.

1. Sensory information usually travels from the _____ nervous system to the _____ nervous system.

2. The nerves that carry information from sensory receptors to the brain and spinal cord are called _____, while those that convey information from the central nervous system to muscles or glands are called _____.

3. The three layers of the meninges in order from deep to superficial are the _____ _____, the _____, and the _____ _____.

4. Brain and spinal cord tissue composed primarily of neurons is referred to as _____ _____ due to the darker pigmentation of its fat component, while the tissue of the central nervous system composed primarily of axons and myelin is called _____ _____.

5. The three developmental divisions of the brain are called the _____, _____, and _____.

6. The four lobes of the cerebral hemispheres are the _____, _____, _____, and _____.

7. The hindbrain consists of three distinct portions called the _____, _____ _____, and _____.

8. The two divisions of the peripheral nervous system are the _____ and _____ branches.

9. Motor nerves stem from the _____ _____ of the spinal cord, while sensory nerves stem from the _____ _____.

10. Cranial and spinal nerves give rise to the _____ division of the _____ nervous system, but the _____ division arises from the thoracic and lumbar regions.

Matching

Match each of the following terms with the clue that best describes it by placing the letter of the term in the blank next to the correct clue.

a) abducens

b) audition

c) central sulcus

d) choroid plexus

e) epineurium

f) glioma

g) gustation

h) hypoglossal

i) insula

j) meninges

k) papillae

l) plasticity

m) rhodopsin

n) ventricles

o) vestibule

_____ neuroglial tumor

_____ site of taste buds

_____ memory processing

_____ brain cavities

_____ detection of body position

_____ brain membrane

_____ result of neuron experience

_____ sensitivity

_____ outer nerve covering

_____ eye movement

_____ hearing

_____ makes cerebrospinal fluid

_____ taste

_____ separates frontal and parietal lobes

_____ tongue movement

Complete the Terms Table

Complete the missing key terms and/or definitions in the following table.

Term	Definition
redundancy	
	a nervous system disorder that causes slow, involuntary movements of the hands and feet
	a tumor that develops from nervous system cells
arteriovenous malformation	
	disorder of blood vessels in the brain
semicircular canals	
	a depression in the retina that contains only cones
	the clear covering at the front surface of the eye that permits light to enter
olfactory bulb	
	cranial nerve that is sensory for transmitting cardiovascular reflexes and has motor control of the heart and digestion

extrapyramidal tract	
	a collection of nuclei at the base of the cerebrum that is associated with emotions
ventricles	
	the cerebral lobe that interprets vision and assists with eye function
	a band of white matter that connects the left and right hemispheres of the cerebrum

Label the Graphic

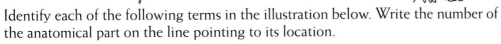

Identify each of the following terms in the illustration below. Write the number of the anatomical part on the line pointing to its location.

1. abducens
2. accessory
3. glossopharyngeal
4. hypoglossal
5. oculomotor
6. olfactory

7. optic
8. trigeminal
9. trochlear
10. vagus
11. vestibular

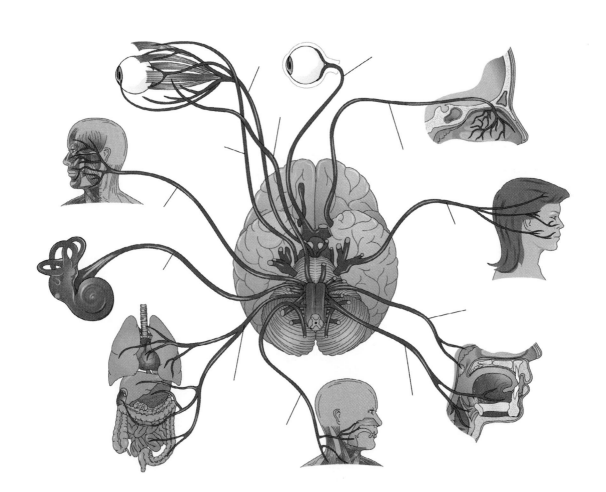

1. Which of the cranial nerves have a sensory function?

2. Which have motor function?

Color the Graphic

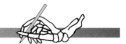

Color this illustration using the following key:

brain stem – orange
central sulcus – black
cerebellum – pink
frontal lobe – blue
lateral fissure – brown
occipital lobe – yellow
parietal lobe – green
temporal lobe – red

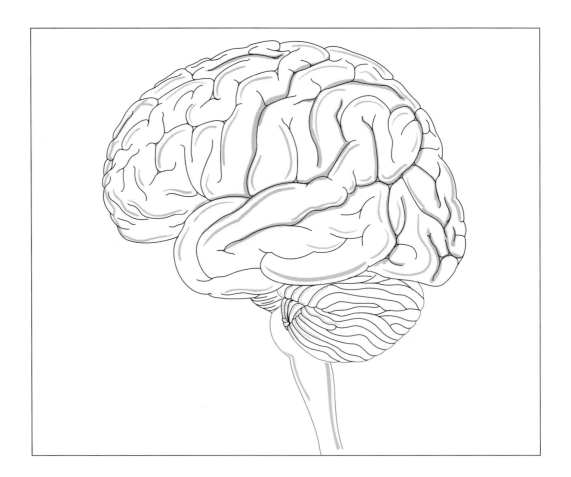

1. The forebrain comprises which parts of the brain?

2. Describe the position of the cerebellum and medulla oblongata in relation to the pons.

3. Which developmental portion of the brain comprises the cerebellum, pons, and medulla oblongata?

4. Which developmental portion of the brain is located between the forebrain and hindbrain.

Practical Application

Write brief responses to the following scenarios.

1. Drugs known as beta blockers are so called because they bind to certain adrenergic (norepinephrine or epinephrine) receptors that are classified as beta type. When this drug binds to beta receptors they can no longer bind to epinephrine and so the normal effects of this neurotransmitter's activity are "blocked." What effect would such a drug have on cardiac activity?

2. The drug cocaine blocks the reuptake of catecholamines at the synaptic cleft. What implication would this have on the user's cardiovascular system?

3. The results of a recent study presented at an American Heart Association meeting was the first to actually show scientific, quantitative data indicating that the use of pet therapy can help the recovery of heart-failure patients. The data included measurement of patients' epinephrine levels. Do you think data that support the use of pet therapy to increase recovery showed an increase or a decrease in epinephrine levels of patients who were visited by dogs during their recovery? Explain how this would aid in recovery.

4. What are some possible physical abnormalities that might occur if a person has suffered damage to the brain stem? Discuss the possibilities in relation to the specific site of damage.

5. A technique recently developed by researchers might make detection of Alzheimer's disease possible before the neuron death associated with the disease occurs. (Currently, Alzheimer's is diagnosed through symptoms but can only be confirmed with 100% certainly through postmortem analysis of the brain tissue.) Alzheimer's disease results from abnormal accumulation of the protein amyloid-beta 42 in brain tissue. The protein is made in all brains, but normally passes into the spinal fluid and is transferred to the blood, where it is filtered out of the body during excretion. The new technique involves monitoring spinal fluid for the presence of this protein. Into which catagory of disease is Alzheimer's catagorized? How would you expect the spinal fluid level of amyloid-beta 42 of a person in the beginning stages of Alzheimer's to compare with that of a person without the disease?

6. What abnormalities might exist from damage to each of the cerebral lobes?

7. To which of the two divisions of the forebrain might improper function of the pituitary gland be attributed, and what is the "connection" between this part of the brain and the endocrine system?

8. What type of sensory receptors most likely detects pheromones, and in which sensory organ(s) would they be located? In addition, what effector might be in a reflex arc response that is elicited by the stimulation of these sensory receptors?

9. How could subarachnoid hemorrhaging could be detected?

10. What advantage does the blood-brain barrier provide for the body? What is a disadvantage that its presence creates in the treatment of certain diseases?

Crossword Puzzle

Complete the following crossword puzzle using key terms from the text.

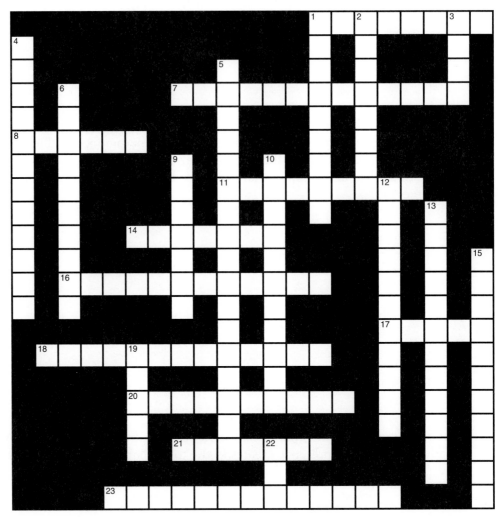

Across

1. blood-vessel swelling
7. detects chemical stimuli
8. gray matter surface of the brain
11. midbrain and hindbrain
14. collections of nerve cells
16. spinal-cord cavity
17. monosodium-glutamate (MSG) taste
18. excess cerebrospinal fluid
20. sensory cranial nerves from face and mouth
21. external ear
23. bundles of nervous-tissue cells

Down

1. sensory-nerve tracts leading to the brain
2. carries information away
3. taste one senses when acids dissolve
4. contains the thalamus and hypo-thalamus
5. sensory cranial nerves for balance and hearing
6. nerve pathway
9. peripheral nerves arising from the brain
10. gray-matter pockets in the brain
12. connective tissue separating nerve cells
13. brain-covering space filled with cere-brospinal fluid
15. left and right halves of the cerebrum
19. sensory cranial nerves for vision
22. the brain and spinal cord

1. Information from the CNS to muscles or glands is carried by:

   a) sensory neurons
   b) afferent neurons
   c) motor neurons
   d) All of the above

2. Which of the following best describes the endoneurium?

   a) separates nerve cells from one another
   b) surrounds axons and myelin
   c) maintains selectivity of what enters and exits axons
   d) All of the above

3. Ganglia of the central nervous system:

   a) are anatomically identical to those of the peripheral nervous system
   b) usually have a motor function
   c) would not have Nodes of Ranvier as part of their anatomy
   d) All of the above

4. Which of the following best describes the meninges?

   a) separate the brain from the skull and the spinal cord from the vertebrae
   b) consist of three distinct layers
   c) are associated with ependymal cells for cerebrospinal fluid production
   d) All of the above

5. Gray matter is composed mainly of _____ and is located
   _____ in the spinal cord:

   a) neurons/centrally
   b) axons/centrally
   c) neurons/peripherally
   d) axons/peripherally

6. Basal nuclei in the brain:

   a) function for memory
   b) function for body movement
   c) relay sensory information to the brain
   d) control emotion

7. Which of the following statements is true of the cerebral hemispheres?

   a) Both are involved equally in determining an individual's behavior.
   b) Specialized regions for speech and language are present in the right hemisphere.
   c) Dominance of the right hemisphere is attributed to artistic talent.
   d) All of the above

8. Damage to the temporal lobe might affect the ability to:

   a) move your legs
   b) focus your eyes correctly
   c) feel hunger
   d) recognize a friend's voice

9. The ventricles of the central nervous system:

   a) are isolated cavities within the brain
   b) circulate cerebrospinal fluid
   c) provide space for air circulation in the brain
   d) All of the above

10. The portion of the brain that plays a major role in autonomic control of breathing and cardiovascular function is the:

    a) medulla oblongata
    b) pons
    c) midbrain
    d) diencephalon

11. A person with degeneration of the cerebellum would most likely experience loss of:

    a) vision
    b) memory
    c) balance
    d) All of the above

12. Ascending nerve tracts:

    a) carry sensory information
    b) carry motor information
    c) are located ventrally in the spinal column
    d) All of the above

13. The cranial nerves are:

    a) part of the central nervous system
    b) part of the peripheral nervous system
    c) surrounded by the meninges and cerebrospinal fluid
    d) solely sensory in function

14. Dorsal root ganglia:

    a) have ascending axons
    b) are located in the ventral horn of gray matter
    c) have motor function
    d) All of the above

15. Which of the following is true about the arrangement of neurons in the autonomic nervous system?

    a) Preganglionic neurons are myelinated, while postganglionic neurons are not.
    b) Preganglionic neurons of the parasympathetic nervous system are long when compared with postganglionic neurons.
    c) Preganglionic neurons of the sympathetic nervous system are short compared to the postganglionic neurons.
    d) All of the above

16. In the autonomic nervous system, postganglionic neurons:

    a) of the parasympathetic system always innervate effectors that are different than those of the sympathetic system
    b) of both the parasympathetic and sympathetic systems secrete the same neurotransmitters
    c) of the sympathetic system secrete norepinephrine
    d) All of the above

17. Acetylcholine is the neurotransmitter secreted by:

    a) parasympathetic postganglionic neurons
    b) preganglionic neurons of both sympathetic and parasympathetic neurons
    c) neurons causing skeletal muscle contraction
    d) All of the above

18. Which of the following statements is true regarding sympathetic nerve activity?

    a) It is always excitatory.
    b) It is always inhibitory.
    c) It is excitatory to some receptors and inhibitory to others.
    d) It is only excitatory to skeletal muscles.

19. Which of the following is a correct pathway for sound transmission?

    a) external auditory meatus, tympanic membrane, malleus, incus, stapes, oval window, and round window
    b) auricle, tympanic membrane, incus, malleus, stapes, oval window, and round window
    c) tympanic membrane, malleus, incus, stapes, round window, and oval window
    d) oval window, tympanic membrane, malleus, incus stapes, and round window

20. Whiplash is an example of a(n):

    a) cerebrovascular disease
    b) traumatic neuropathy
    c) arteriovenous malformation
    d) neurodegenerative disease

21. Aneurysms, arteriovenous malformations, and ischemic attacks are all examples of:

    a) neurodegenerative disease
    b) traumatic neuropathy
    c) effects of aging
    d) vascular anomalies

22. Which of the following nervous system disorders is the result of abnormal dopamine production?

    a) chorea
    b) palsy
    c) athetosis
    d) All of the above

23. Decreased function of sensory perception in elderly persons is most likely attributed to:

    a) the extreme loss of neurons that accompanies aging
    b) plasticity and/or redundancy
    c) degradation of the sensory structures
    d) All of the above

24. Plasticity and redundancy:

    a) are compensatory mechanisms of aging
    b) have a direct correlation with dendrite number
    c) are increased by regular mental and physical activity throughout the lifetime
    d) All of the above

25. Match the letter of each of the following clues with its corresponding sense. Letters may be used more than once.

    a) audition   _____ conjunctiva

    b) equilibrium   _____ tympanic membrane

    c) gustation   _____ chemoreceptors

    d) olfaction   _____ ciliary body

    e) vision   _____ smell

                    _____ sclera

                    _____ taste buds

                    _____ retina

                    _____ lacrimal

                    _____ eustachian tube

                    _____ cochlea

                    _____ vestibule

10 THE RESPIRATORY SYSTEM

Completion

Complete the following sentences by filling in each blank with a key term from the text.

1. The part of the respiratory system that comprises the nose, nasal cavity, paranasal sinuses, eustachian tubes, and larynx is the _____ _____ system, while the trachea, bronchial tree, and lungs are considered the _____ _____ system.

2. The network of passages that supply the lungs with air is called the _____ _____. Is composed of the right and left _____, which continually branch to form _____ _____, _____ _____, _____, and _____ _____.

3. The upper part of the throat behind the nose is referred to as the _____; it contains the immune system structures called _____, while the part of the throat just inferior is called the _____; it contains the immune system structures known as the _____.

4. The three major cartilages that form the larynx are the _____, _____, and _____.

5. The _____ is the serous membrane of the lungs; it consists of the inner _____ layer and the outer _____ layer.

6. Breathing is often referred to as _____, further differentiated as either _____, which describes the mechanical process of breathing, or _____, which means the exchange of oxygen and carbon dioxide between the blood and body cells.

7. Air movement into the lungs, known as _____, occurs when the diaphragm _____. _____, or movement of air out of the lung, occurs when the diaphragm relaxes.

8. Inflammation caused by infection in only one lobe of the lung is called
   _____ _____, but widespread, infectious inflammation is
   called _____.

9. A common viral disease spread through respiratory fluids is _____.
   A rare viral respiratory disease that can be contracted through rodent contact
   is _____ _____, (_____).

10. The maximum quantity of air the lungs can hold after forced breathing is a
    measurement called _____ _____ _____; it is the
    the sum of the measurements _____ _____ and
    _____ _____.

Matching

Match each of the following terms with the clue that best describes it by placing the
letter of the term in the blank next to the correct clue.

a) atelectasis

b) bronchodilation

c) diaphragm

d) emphysema

e) Heimlich maneuver

f) intrapleural pressure

g) laryngeal prominence

h) larynx

i) lobule

j) nares

k) pharynx

l) restrictive lung disease

m) tidal volume

n) ventilation

o) vomeronasal gland

_____ alveoli damage

_____ choking

_____ the nostrils

_____ the throat

_____ prevents lung collapse

_____ chemoreceptors

_____ voice box

_____ inadequate lung expansion

_____ lung collapse

_____ breathing

_____ Adam's apple

_____ respiratory passage enlargement

_____ breathing muscle

_____ a normal breath

_____ subdivision of the lungs

Complete the Terms Table

Complete the missing key terms and/or definitions in the following table.

Term	Definition
	air cavities within the facial bones
trachea	
epiglottis	
	the constriction of smooth-muscle bands in the terminal bronchioles
alveolus	
partial pressure	
	the abnormal stretching and dilation of the bronchi or bronchioles
	a lung infection caused by the inactive stage of a worm
Acute Respiratory Distress Syndrome (ARDS)	
	the amount of air moved into and out of the lungs in one minute
inspiratory reserve volume	
	the amount of air that is forcefully expired after a normal exhalation

Label the Graphic

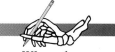

Identify each of the following terms in the illustration on page 110. Write the number of the anatomical part on the line pointing to its location.

1. alveolar duct
2. alveolar sac
3. alveoli
4. bronchioles
5. capillary
6. laryngopharynx
7. larynx
8. left and right primary bronchi
9. lower respiratory tract
10. lungs
11. nasal cavity
12. nasopharynx
13. oropharynx
14. trachea
15. upper respiratory tract

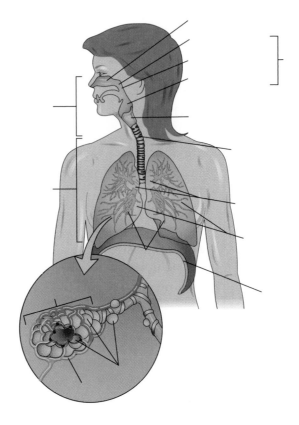

1. Beginning with the nasal cavity, the lining of the respiratory tract has special hairlike structures and a layer of a substance secreted by the epithelial cells. What are the names of these two components of the tract lining, and what purpose do they serve?

2. Where does gas exchange between the air and lungs actually take place?

3. Why does the left lung have a notch at its inferior medial end?

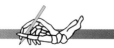

Color the Graphic

Color this illustration using the following color key:

adenoids – light green
parnasal sinuses – brown
tonsils – dark green
nasopharynx – yellow
oropharynx – orange
laryngopharynx – red
epiglottis – light blue
thyroid cartilage – dark blue
vocal cords – black
trachea – pink

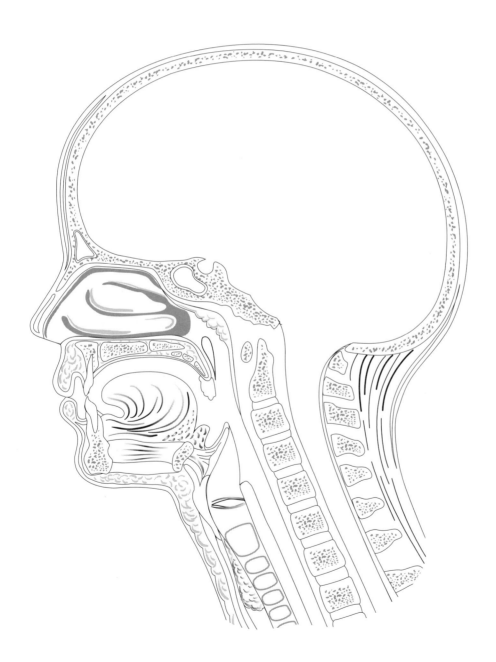

111

Practical Application

Write brief responses to the following scenarios.

1. Cigarette smoking causes the movement of the cilia lining the respiratory tract to cease. What connection does this have with the excessive coughing that is characteristic of a smoker?

2. Cystic fibrosis is a genetic disease that causes a drastic increase in the amount of mucus produced in the body. It is common for the bronchioles to become blocked in this disease state. What type of damage would probably occur and what is the term used to describe this condition?

3. Why might someone experience soreness in the chest following heavy aerobic exercise? Include more specific locations of soreness in your answer.

4. Breathing is under involuntarily control of the nervous system. The initial need to increase the breathing rate and depth is detected by a buildup of carbon dioxide in the blood (detected in the brain as the increase in hydrogen ion content resulting) rather than a lack of oxygen. What type of receptors would detect this stimulus? What specific division of the nervous system would be involved? What would be the effectors in the reflex arc? What could a runner voluntarily do to help keep the increased need for breathing rate to a minimum?

5. What affect do you think breathing into a paper bag would have on the partial pressure of oxygen and carbon dioxide in the blood versus the atmosphere?

6. How might a stab wound to the thorax interrupt mechanical breathing even if it were not deep enough to actually enter the lung?

7. What is it about the anatomy of the lungs that prevents damage in one location from having a detrimental effect on other lung locations?

8. Which division of the nervous system would be activated by drugs used to treat asthma?

9. Although about 30% of the carbon dioxide in the blood is transported by binding to red blood cells, the majority of these molecules are converted to a compound called carbonic acid which quickly dissociates into bicarbonate ions and hydrogen ions. How is this significant in the respiratory system's role in body homeostatis? Give an example of another body system that could be affected.

10. While having dinner with a friend, a woman appears to have trouble swallowing and clearly tells you that she thinks she is choking. Should you consider performing the Heimlich maneuver?

Crossword Puzzle

Complete the following crossword puzzle using key terms from the text.

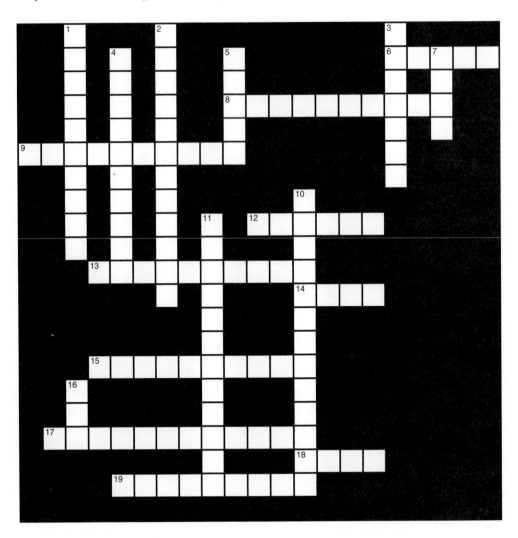

Across

6. organs of gas exchange
8. inflammation of the bronchi
9. sound-producing muscles
12. vocal cord location
13. inspiration
14. persistent obstruction of bronchial air-flow
15. clean and moisten air
17. *Mycobacterium* bacteria
18. unit of pressure measurement
19. lung membrane inflammation

Down

1. reduces lung water evaporation
2. air in the pleural cavity
3. the larynx opening
4. expiration
5. lung subdivision
7. respiratory entryway
10. treated with bronchodilators
11. nose cartilage
16. short for influenza

1. The exchange of gas between the respiratory and circulatory systems occurs by:

   a) active transport
   b) osmosis
   c) passive diffusion
   d) All of the above

2. Which of the following respiratory components can be considered a part of either the upper or lower respiratory tract?

   a) eustachian tube
   b) pharynx
   c) trachea
   d) larynx

3. The purpose of the large number of blood vessels in the nasal cavity is to:

   a) moisten the air
   b) warm the air
   c) transfer gases
   d) remove foreign material

4. The paranasal cavities:

   a) lighten the skull
   b) function in speech resonance
   c) warm and moisten air
   d) All of the above

5. In what other body system is the pharynx also a component?

   a) lymphatic
   b) muscular
   c) digestive
   d) endocrine

6. Incomplete closure of which structure can allow food to accidentally enter the respiratory passages?

   a) epiglottis
   b) thyroid cartilage
   c) larynx
   d) glottis

7. The vocal cords are muscles housed by the _____ and held in place by the _____.

   a) pharynx/cricoid cartilage
   b) larynx/epiglottis
   c) pharynx/arytenoid cartilage
   d) larynx/arytenoid cartilage

8. Which of the following best describes the trachea?

    a) contains circular tracheal cartilages
    b) is anterior to the esophagus
    c) functions for gas exchange with the blood
    d) All of the above

9. Which of the following best describes the bronchioles?

    a) are smaller than bronchi
    b) contain no cartilage
    c) control air volume by constricting and dilating smooth muscle
    d) All of the above

10. Sympathetic nerve innervation would _____ air intake by _____.

    a) increase/bronchodilation
    b) increase/bronchoconstriction
    c) decrease/bronchocontriction
    d) decrease/bronchodilation

11. Damage in one area of the lung:

    a) prevents the proper function of the complete organ
    b) is usually a life-threatening situation
    c) affects all lobes
    d) is localized by the independent functioning of lobes and lobules

12. Which of the following best describes the action of surfactant in the lungs?

    a) catalyzes gas exchange
    b) engulfs microbes
    c) prevents evaporation and alveolar collapse
    d) All of the above

13. Where in the lungs does gas exchange occur?

    a) in the alveoli
    b) in the respiratory portion of the lobules
    c) across epithelial cells
    d) All of the above

14. Oxygen and carbon dioxide gas exhange:

    a) always occurs as a result of breathing
    b) depends on the partial pressures of each gas
    c) is often referred to as external respiration
    d) All of the above

15. Breathing is under:

    a) involuntary control
    b) voluntary control
    c) sympathetic and parasympathetic control
    d) All of the above

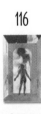

16. When the diaphragm contracts, it:

    a) forces air out of the lungs
    b) lowers
    c) increases the internal pressure of the lungs
    d) All of the above

17. Air moves into the lungs due to:

    a) a decrease in lung volume
    b) an increase in the thoracic-cavity pressure
    c) a decrease in the thoracic-cavity pressure
    d) relaxation of the diaphragm

18. Relaxation of the diaphragm causes:

    a) a decrease in lung volume
    b) an increase in thoracic pressure
    c) upward movement of the diaphragm
    d) All of the above

19. The difference in gas levels between the air in the alveoli and the alveolar capillary blood:

    a) controls the measurement known as partial pressure
    b) controls mechanical breathing
    c) establishes active transport measures
    d) All of the above

20. If the partial pressure of a gas is higher in the blood than in the atmosphere, that gas:

    a) will remain in the blood
    b) will leave the blood
    c) is present in a higher concentration in the atmosphere
    d) will not diffuse across the alveolar membrane

21. How does the partial pressure of carbon dioxide in the blood entering the alveoli normally compare with the atmospheric partial pressure of carbon dioxide?

    a) It is higher.
    b) It is lower.
    c) It is equivalent.
    d) It consistently fluctuates from higher to lower.

22. Atelectasis could result from:

    a) chronic obstructive pulmonary disease (COPD)
    b) pneumothorax
    c) lung cancer
    d) All of the above

23. Which of the following would result in bronchiectasis?

   a) asthma
   b) bronchitis
   c) long-term accumulation of mucus
   d) All of the above

24. Which of the following is an example of an infectious respiratory disease?

   a) tuberculosis
   b) pneumonia
   c) influenza
   d) All of the above

25. Which of the following measurements of lung capacity reflects the fact that the lungs are never totally empty of air?

   a) tidal volume
   b) vital capacity
   c) residual volume
   d) expiratory reserve volume

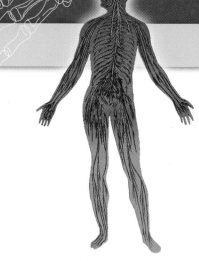

THE CARDIOVASCULAR SYSTEM

Completion

Complete the following sentences by filling in each blank with a key term from the text.

1. _____ is a term used to describe the development and growth of blood vessels. It is directed by chemicals called _____ _____.

2. The three major types of vessels that transport blood are _____, _____, and _____.

3. Arteries and veins have three distinct layers: the inner _____, middle _____, and outer _____.

4. The _____ side of the heart pumps blood to the body, which is known as _____ circulation, and the _____ side pumps blood to the _____, or into _____ circulation.

5. _____ _____, or lack of oxygen in the heart, can cause the heart to function abnormally and lead to muscle cell death or _____ _____ if severe enough.

6. The valves separating the upper and lower heart chambers are the _____; the one on the left is the _____, or _____, and the one on the right is the _____. The valves separating each ventricle from the blood vessels that leave the heart are the _____.

7. The heart's electrical conduction is initiated by the _____ _____, and continues in a specific order to the _____ _____, the _____, and the _____ _____.

8. In the fetal heart, an opening between the right and left atria called the _____ _____ and a blood vessel between the pulmonary artery and the aorta called the _____ _____ allow blood to bypass the lungs.

9. One complete contraction and relaxation of the heart is called the
_____ _____. It consists of two stages: 1) _____,
which is heart muscle relaxation and ventricular filling; and 2)
_____, which is ventricular contraction and ejection of blood.

10. The medical terms for the progressive narrowing and hardening of arteries
due to _____ formation are often differentiated as resulting from fat
deposits called _____ or calcium deposits called _____.

Matching

Match each of the following terms with the clue that best describes it by placing the
letter of the term in the blank next to the correct clue.

a) aneurysm   _____ pericardial visceral layer

b) aorta   _____ blood clot

c) atrium   _____ blood-vessel bulge

d) cardiac output   _____ upper heart chamber

e) coronary artery   _____ rapid cardiac muscle contraction

f) epicardium   _____ diameter decrease

g) fibrillation   _____ vein branch

h) myocardium   _____ amount of blood pumped by the heart
                                 each minute

i) prolapse   _____ exits the left ventricle

j) pulmonary artery   _____ lower heart chamber

k) SA node   _____ stretched heart valve

l) thrombosis   _____ starts the heart beat

m) vasoconstriction   _____ exits the right ventricle

n) ventricle   _____ cardiac muscle

o) venules   _____ supplies blood to the heart muscle

Complete the Terms Table

Complete the missing key terms and/or definitions in the following table.

Term	Definition
	the widening of the diameter of a blood vessel
pericardium	
	specialized muscle cells that carry the electric impulses through the ventricles
papillary muscles	
venae cavae	
	the amount of blood the ventricle of the heart pumps with each beat
electrocardiography	
	the portion of an electrocardiogram that represents ventricular depolarization and contraction
	dhest pain due to coronary heart disease
endocarditis	
	irregular rhythmic beating of the heart
	a condition in which the heart cannot pump out all of the blood that enters the chambers
	heart valve damage due to *Streptococcus* bacterial infection
cardiovagal baroreflex	
sudden cardiac death	

Label the Graphic

Identify each of the following terms in the illustration on page 122. Write the number of the anatomical part on the line pointing to its location.

1. aortic semilunar valve
2. bicuspid valve
3. chordae tendinae
4. inferior vena cava
5. interventricular septum
6. left atrium
7. left ventricle
8. papillary muscle
9. pulmonary artery
10. pulmonary semilunar valve
11. pulmonary veins
12. right atrium
13. right ventricle
14. superior vena cava
15. tricuspid valve

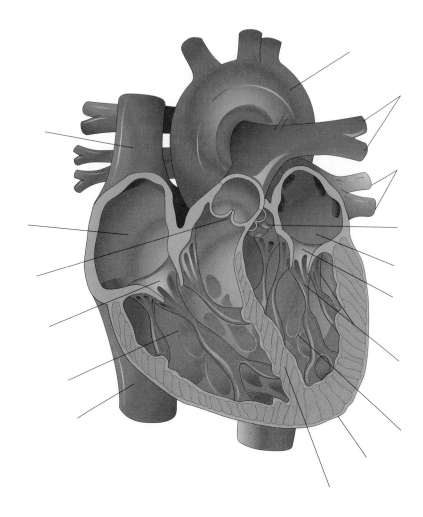

1. Is the blood in the pulmonary arteries high or low in oxygen content?

2. Which side of the heart sends blood into systemic circulation?

3. Which side of the heart receives blood from pulmonary circulation?

4. Which side of the heart receives blood that is low in oxygen content?

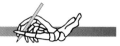

Color the Graphic

Color this illustration using the following color key:

superior vena cava – red
right atrium – pink
left atrium – green
right ventricle – yellow
left ventricle – purple
inferior vena cava – brown
interventricular septum – blue
aorta – orange

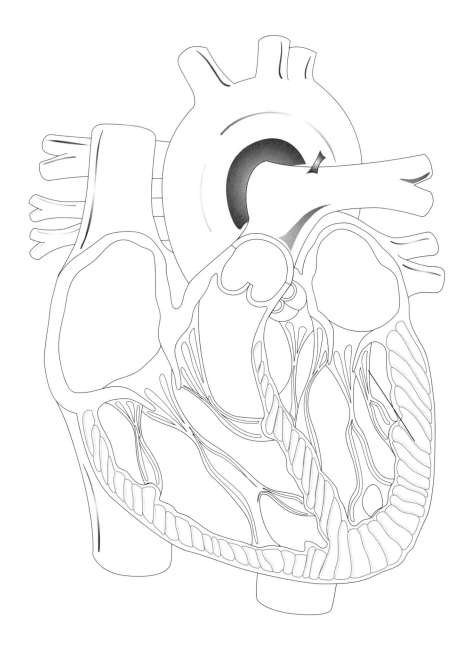

Practical Application

Write brief responses to the following scenarios.

1. The heart is often described as a "dual pump." Give an explanation for this description. Include in your answer the oxygen and carbon dioxide gas levels of blood.

2. Give a reason why a person would most likely feel more "tired" after standing still for long periods of time than if he or she had been leisurely walking.

3. Plasma and the interstitial fluid have essentially the same composition under normal body homeostasis with the exception of protein levels. The interstitial fluid contains very little protein. Why?

4. The water component of plasma leaves the blood stream to enter tissue by the process of filtration and is reabsorbed by osmosis. Where does each of these processes for water movement between the blood and interstitial space occur, and why does water exit by filtration but reenter by osmosis? What is the significance of the protein imbalance between plasma and interstitial fluid to water movement?

5. Assuming that the total length of the arteries in the body is approximately the same as the total length of the veins, in which of these vessel types is there more blood and why?

6. What is the connection to the cardiovascular system when skin turns red during periods of physical exertion?

7. One cause of a heart murmur is weakening of the chordae tendinae brought on by tissue damage from bacterial infection. What is the name of a disease with this pathology, and what is the anatomical and mechanical connection between the weakened chordae tendinae and a heart murmur?

8. Why does blood in the right side of the fetal heart mix with blood on its left side, and why does this pose no problem for the fetus while it would create a dangerous situation following birth?

9. An abnormal delay in the electrical conduction from the AV node to the bundle of His would affect what phase of the cardiac cycle? At what point of the ECG wave pattern would this be detectable?

10. The constriction of the arteries in a hypertensive state creates a higher-than-normal resistance to the blood being ejected into the aorta following ventricular contraction. Therefore, less blood is able to exit the ventricle than would be ejected in a nonhypertensive state. How would this affect cardiac output? Explain how the body could compensate to maintain normal cardiac output.

Crossword Puzzle

Complete the following crossword puzzle using key terms from the text.

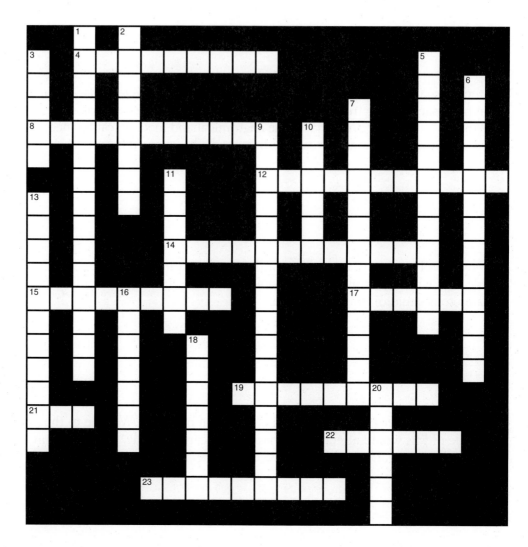

Across

4. ventricular contractions per minute
8. heart epithelial lining
12. another name for the cardiovascular system
14. pericardium inflammation
15. accompanies arterial aging
17. electrical relay between heart chambers
19. obstructs chamber filling
21. measures heart electrical activity
22. innermost pericardium layer
23. right semilunar valve

Down

1. attach papillary muscles and AV valves
2. chronically stretched or dilated
3. interior space
5. high blood pressure
6. can result from obesity and excessive exercise
7. backflow
9. flow of small volumes of blood
10. abnormal heart sound
11. difficult breathing
13. having openings for material exchange
16. outermost pericardium layer
18. heart rate that decreases with age
20. left semilunar valve

Quiz

1. Which of the following would be false regarding pulse and blood pressure?

   a) a pulse is detectable because of blood pressure
   b) an increase in pulse always indicates an increase in blood pressure.
   c) pulse is an indication of the heart rate
   d) blood pressure is a measure of the force of the blood on the blood vessels

2. Which of the following blood vessels carry blood high in oxygen content?
   a) all arteries
   b) all veins
   c) pulmonary arteries
   d) systemic arteries

3. What effect would dehydration have on the hydrostatic pressure of blood?
   a) it would cause it to increase
   b) it would cause it to decrease
   c) it would cause it to fluctuate rapidly
   d) it would have no effect

4. Which of the three layers of blood vessels differs the most between arteries and veins?
   a) tunica media
   b) tunica intima
   c) tunica adventitia
   d) All differ equally

5. Contraction of arterial muscles:
   a) occurs in the tunica media
   b) is called vasoconstriction
   c) narrows the lumen
   d) All of the above

6. Exchange of material between the blood and the body occurs in:
   a) capillaries
   b) arterioles
   c) veins
   d) All of the above

7. Fenestrated capillaries would be least likely to be found in the:
   a) brain
   b) kidneys
   c) small intestines
   d) pituitary gland

8. Which of the following is true about the atria of the heart?
   a) They receive blood.
   b) They exchange blood with one another.
   c) They contain blood high in oxygen.
   d) All of the above

9. Which of the following is true about the ventricles of the heart?
   a) they are completely emptied during systole
   b) they fill with blood during diastole
   c) they contain blood high in oxygen
   d) All of the above

10. Pericardial fluid is contained within which of the following membrane layers surrounding the heart?
    a) myocardium and epicardium
    b) serous pericardium and fibrous pericardium
    c) fibrous pericardium and epicardium
    d) All of the above

11. Coronary blood vessels:
    a) supply the myocardium with blood
    b) consist of arteries high in oxygen and veins low in oxygen
    c) can cause cardiac infarction if blocked
    d) All of the above

12. Which of the following is not true about the AV valves?
    a) they operate through direct sympathetic enervation
    b) they prevent backflow of blood into the atria
    c) the left is called the bicuspid and the right is called the tricuspid
    d) their abnormal stretching is called a prolapse

13. Semilunar valves:
    a) prevent backflow of blood into the ventricles
    b) are forced open as a result of ventricular contraction
    c) are also called the aortic and pulmonary valves
    d) All of the above

14. The right side of the heart:
    a) sends blood into pulmonary circulation
    b) contains blood high in oxygen
    c) contracts with more force than the left side
    d) All of the above

15. An artificial pacemaker replaces the function of which of the following collections of cardiac muscle cells?
    a) bundle of His
    b) purkinje fibers
    c) SA node
    d) AV node

16. An average normal resting heart rate is:
    a) 50 bpm
    b) 75 bpm
    c) 90 bpm
    d) 120 bpm

17. Which of the following sequences is they correct pathway of electrical conduction in the heart?
    a) AV node, SA node, bundle of His, Purkinje system
    b) SA node, AV node, Purkinje system, bundle of His
    c) SA node, AV node, bundle of His, Purkinje system
    d) Sa node, bundle of His, AV node, Purkinje system

18. The ductus arteriosis:
    a) provides the fetal lungs with oxygen
    b) separates the right and left fetal heart atria
    c) provides a bypass for blood from the fetal lungs
    d) All of the above

19. The QRS complex of the ECG
    a) represents ventricular depolarization and contraction.
    b) would be widened by a delay in electrical conduction by the bundle of His.
    c) corresponds with ventricular systole.
    d) All of the above

20. The distance from the beginning of one P wave to the beginning of the next P wave:
    a) is called the P-R interval
    b) would correspond to one complete contraction and relaxation of the heart
    c) would decrease with a slowing heartbeat
    d) can be used to measure blood pressure

21. Diastole occurs as a result of:
    a) atrial depolarization
    b) ventricular filling
    c) atrial contraction
    d) ventricular relaxation

22. Which of the following best describes congestive heart failure?
    a) more than the normal amount of blood remains in the ventricles following systole
    b) body tissues do not receive adequate oxygen
    c) blood enters the heart faster than it can be pumped out
    d) All of the above

23. Fibrillation is an example of:
    a) thrombosis
    b) arrhythmia
    c) hypertrophy
    d) aneurysm

24. A heart valve prolapse is associated with:

   a) blood regurgitation
   b) heart murmur
   c) reduced blood-pumping capacity
   d) All of the above

25. Which of the following is not a normal effect of aging on the cardiovascular system?

   a) arterial stiffness
   b) decreased maximal heart rate
   c) varicose veins
   d) decreased cardiovagal baroreflex

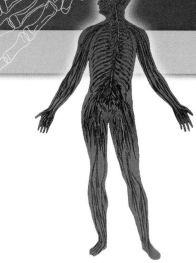

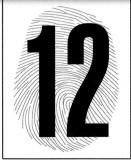

12 THE LYMPHATIC SYSTEM AND THE BLOOD

Completion

Complete the following sentences by filling in each blank with a key term from the text.

1. Blood is composed of a fluid matrix called _____ and three types of cellular components: red blood cells or _____, white blood cells or _____, and _____ also known as _____.

2. The _____ system makes and transports _____ to fight infection.

3. There are three types of white blood cells known as _____: _____, _____, and _____, and two types of white blood cells known as _____: _____ and _____.

4. Blood cells, which are derived from a stem-cell type called _____ or _____, develop into either a white-blood-cell producer or _____ _____, or a red blood cell, platelet, and circulating white-blood-cell producer called a _____ _____.

5. The structural components of the lymphatic system include the lymphatic _____, _____, _____, _____, _____, and _____ blood cells.

6. The immune system responds to disease using two mechanisms: _____ immunity, which is _____ and includes barriers to infection, and _____ immunity, which is very specific and responds in two stages: the _____ _____, which is the initial response to an antigen, and the _____ response, which occurs upon a subsequent exposure to the same antigen.

7. When macrophages attach to _____-lymphocytes they produce _____ _____ that make antibodies or _____, as well as _____ _____ that store the information to produce antibodies.

131

8. The immunity that results from antibody production by B-lymphocytes is called _____ _____, while immunity resulting from intact cells—primarily T-lymphocytes—is called _____ _____.

9. Immunity against disease can be acquired through _____ immunity, which is gained by exposure to foreign antigens or _____ immunity, which requires the introduction of antibodies.

10. Various types of _____ result from deficiency of red blood cells; insufficient vitamin B12 causes _____ _____; a genetic disorder called _____ _____ causes a type of _____ or abnormal hemoglobin disorder; and the presence of abnormally large or abnormally small red blood cells causes _____ and _____ _____ respectively.

Matching

Match each of the following terms with the clue that best describes it by placing the letter of the term in the blank next to the correct clue.

a) antigens

b) basophils

c) B-lymphocytes

d) circulating monocytes

e) eosinophils

f) erythropoiesis

g) fibrin

h) hematocrit

i) mast cell

j) megakaryocytes

k) MCHC

l) plasmin

m) prostacyclin

n) red pulp

o) Rh factor

_____ prevents platelet activation

_____ spleen RBC storage removal

_____ packed red cell volume

_____ induce immune response

_____ bone marrow platelet producer

_____ dissolves blood clots

_____ average RBC hemoglobin concentration

_____ antibody production

_____ histamine secretion

_____ blood clot formation

_____ type-D RBC protein

_____ phagocytic blood cells

_____ major basic protein

_____ associated with inflammation

_____ red blood cell formation

Complete the Terms Table

Complete the missing key terms and/or definitions in the following table.

Term	Definition
	a protein in red blood cells that carries oxygen
reticulocyte	
mean corpuscular volume (MCV)	
	the mass of hemoglobin molecules in each red blood cell
	a classification system for the proteins on human red blood cells
carbonic anhydrase	
	an enzyme that stimulates blood clotting by converting fibrinogen into fibrin
Peyer's patches	
	a region of the spleen composed of lymphatic tissue
	a group of innate immunity plasma proteins that can be activated to destroy microorganisms
antibody	
	a T-lymphocyte that inhibits the immune response
	therapeutic exposure to foreign antigens
hemophilia	
	a condition in which the body produces an immune response against its own organs or tissues

Label the Graphic

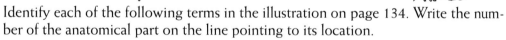

Identify each of the following terms in the illustration on page 134. Write the number of the anatomical part on the line pointing to its location.

1. B-lymphocyte
2. basophil
3. eosinophil
4. lymphoid stem cell
5. macrophage
6. megakaryocyte
7. monocyte
8. myeloid stem cell
9. neutrophil
10. plasma cell
11. platelets
12. pre-B cell
13. pre-T cell
14. red blood cell
15. reticulocyte
16. T-lymphocyte
17. tissue mast cell

pluripotential stem cell

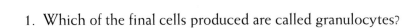

1. Which of the final cells produced are called granulocytes?

2. Which of the final cells produced are called agranulocytes?

3. Which of the final components of blood lack nuclei?

Color the Graphic

Color this illustration using the following color key:

axillary lymph nodes – dark blue
cervical lymph nodes – green
inguinal lymph nodes – yellow
lymph vessels of the lumbar trunk – highlight in yellow
popliteal lymph nodes – black
spleen – red
submandibular lymph nodes – brown
thoracic duct – highlight in pink
thymus – light blue
tonsils – orange

1. What are the three components of lymph nodes?

2. What is the name of the location of a lymph node where the blood vessels enter and lymphatic vessels exit?

3. What is the name of the fluid-filled sac within a lymph node?

4. What is the name of the capsular wall partitions within a lymph node that create regions housing B- and T-cell lymphocytes?

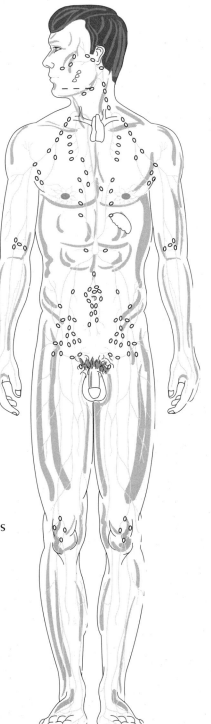

THE LYMPHATIC SYSTEM AND THE BLOOD

Practical Application

Write brief responses to the following scenarios.

1. Is it always a good idea to immediately treat a mild fever with fever-reducing medication? Why or why not?

2. What effect would dehydration of the body have on a hematocrit reading and why?

3. Would it be possible for an individual to have had a malignancy at some point in his or her lifetime that no longer exists and to have had no knowledge of its existence? Explain.

4. The lower oxygen content of air at high elevations causes an increase in red blood cell production. How would this affect blood viscosity, and what problem might this pose for an individual with hypertension?

5. Of what importance is the vasodilatory effect of histamine in the immune response?

6. The condition called jaundice exists when bilirubin accumulates in the blood plasma and causes the yellow appearance of the skin and whites of the eyes. This chemical is normally removed from the body by the liver and digestive system. What connection is there between blood and bilirubin? Assuming that the liver and digestive system are properly functioning to remove bilirubin, what abnormality might jaundice indicate about the individual's blood?

7. What pathological condition is indicated by interferon production by a cell?

8. Compare and contrast the immune system's role in the spleen and lymph nodes.

9. A dangerous practice used by some athletes called "blood doping" involves injecting commercially prepared erythropoietin into the body prior to an athletic competition. What do you suppose is the benefit being sought by these athletes and what is dangerous about this practice?

10. The blood of a mother and fetus does not normally "mix" with the exception that some of the fetal blood can actually leak into the mother's blood at the very late stage of pregnancy or during birth. What risk factor would this pose in a situation where the woman is Rh negative but the child is Rh positive? To whom does the risk factor belong? Could this affect subsequent pregnancies? (NOTE: Although fetal and maternal blood do not normally mix, antibodies are small enough to diffuse through the maternal and fetal circulatory membranes.)

Crossword Puzzle

Complete the following crossword puzzle using key terms from the text.

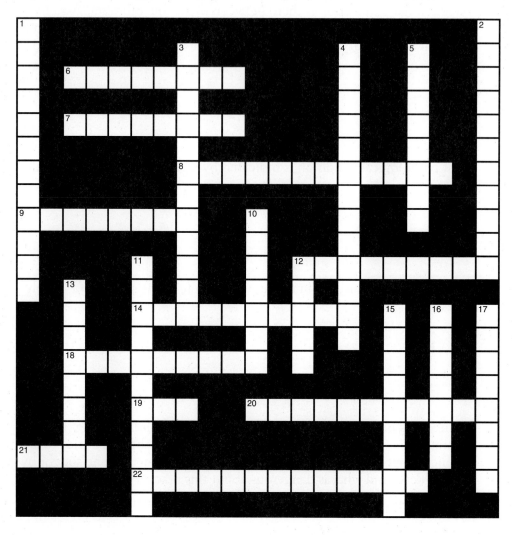

Across

6. cancer that elevates white blood cell count
7. of moderate duration
8. immune response of swelling, redness, warmth, or pain
9. Hodgkin's and non-Hodgkin's cancer
12. result from immune hypersensitivity
14. separates cells from plasma
18. RBC protein classification
19. virus that causes AIDS
20. phagocytic liver monocyte
21. immature white blood cell
22. lymphedema caused by parasitic infection

Down

1. immature red blood cell
2. bacteria-killing chemicals
3. builds acquired immune response
4. tumor-killing T-lymphocytes
5. complete blood cell count
10. antigen-containing drug
11. tissue monocytes
12. sudden or severe
13. injected antibody-like protein
15. produced from hemoglobin breakdown
16. red-blood-cell-bound antigen
17. disease of Jenner's vaccine studies

Quiz

1. Which of the following distinguishes blood from other connective-tissue types?

   a) it supports other body tissues
   b) it contains cells and a matrix
   c) it has a fluid matrix
   d) its cells are in a dispersed arrangement

2. Which of the following cellular components would not be considered "complete" cells?

   a) erythrocytes
   b) thrombocytes
   c) platelets
   d) All of the above

3. Which of the following values of a CBC would be expressed in %?

   a) hematocrit
   b) MCV
   c) MCH
   d) All of the above

4. A person with type O blood:

   a) could be a recipient of all other blood types
   b) could be a donor for all other blood types
   c) has protein called type O on the red blood cells
   d) All of the above

5. Erythroblastosis fetalis occurs when:

   a) a mother and her developing fetus have incompatible ABO blood types
   b) when either the mother or developing fetus is Rh positive and the other is Rh negative
   c) when a mother is Rh negative and her developing fetus is Rh positive
   d) All of the above

6. In a normal differential white blood cell count the highest percentage of cells would be:

   a) neutrophils
   b) erythrocytes
   c) lymphocytes
   d) eosinophils

7. A patient with a parasitic infection would probably have an abnormally high count of:

   a) erythrocytes
   b) monocytes
   c) neutrophils
   d) eosinophils

8. Which of the following is not a granulocyte?
   a) eosinophil
   b) basophil
   c) lymphocyte
   d) neutrophil

9. How many molecules of oxygen would be carried per cubic millimeter of blood in a person with a normal red blood cell count?
   a) 4 million
   b) 20 million
   c) 120,000
   d) 1 billion

10. Which of the following is not a function of red blood cells?
    a) oxygen transport to tissue
    b) carbon dioxide transport to the lungs
    c) stimulation of bicarbonate-ion formation
    d) immune response

11. Monocytes in tissue are phagocytic cells called:
    a) mast cells
    b) macrophages
    c) basic protein cells
    d) microglia

12. Which of the following represents a correct sequence in clot formation and destruction?
    a) platelet adhesion, fibrinogen, fibrin, plasminogen, and plasmin
    b) plasminogen, plasmin, platelet adhesion, prothrombin, and thrombin
    c) prothrombin, thrombin, plasminogen, plasmin, and clot dissolving
    d) platelet adhesion, prothrombin, thrombin, fibrinogen, and fibrin

13. What type of cell is not produced by bone-marrow myeloid progenitor cells?
    a) platelet
    b) lymphocyte
    c) macrophage
    d) erythrocyte

14. Which of the following is not a component of the lymphatic system?
    a) thyroid
    b) thymus
    c) spleen
    d) leukocytes

15. The removal of red blood cells is accomplished by:
    a) the thymus
    b) white pulp of the spleen
    c) red pulp of the spleen
    d) All of the above

16. Which of the following is not an agent of innate immunity?
    a) skin
    b) complements
    c) natural killer cells
    d) helper T-cells

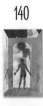

17. The primary response of acquired immunity involves:
    a) macrophage phagocytosis of an antigen
    b) B-lymphocyte division into plasma cells and memory cells
    c) antibody production by B-lymphocytes
    d) All of the above

18. The elevation of this antibody could indicate an allergic reaction:
    a) IgM
    b) IgE
    c) IgD
    d) IgA

19. A vaccine that induces active immunity works by introducing _____ into the body.
    a) antibodies
    b) antibiotics
    c) antigens
    d) All of the above

20. Breast-feeding provides an infant with:
    a) antigens
    b) globulins
    c) antibodies
    d) All of the above

21. Which of the following would not be a cause of anemia?:
    a) high altitude
    b) iron deficiency
    c) internal bleeding
    d) kidney damage

22. A major symptom of lymph vessel blockage is:
    a) fever
    b) swelling
    c) paralysis
    d) anemia

23. HIV causes AIDS by attacking:
    a) B-lymphocytes
    b) suppressor T-cells
    c) helper T-cells
    d) All of the above

24. Which of the following is not associated with hypersensitivity?
    a) IgE antibodies
    b) major basic protein
    c) mast cells
    d) histamine

25. Which of the following is associated with the reduced red blood cell production that accompanies aging?
    a) diminished nutrient absorption
    b) presence of fewer bone marrow stem cells
    c) decrease in kidney erythropoietin
    d) All of the above

141

CHAPTER

THE DIGESTIVE SYSTEM

Completion

Complete the following sentences by filling in each blank with a key term from the text.

1. The digestive system is composed of two components: the _____ _____ or _____ _____ and the _____ _____ _____.

2. The accessory digestive organs include the _____ _____, _____, _____, and _____ _____.

3. The four major types of teeth, beginning with the center position and moving laterally and posteriorly, are the _____, _____, _____, and _____.

4. The four tissue layers making up the esophagus and the rest of the alimentary canal from deep to superficial are the _____ _____, _____, _____, and _____ (_____).

5. The three regions of the stomach (as well as their respective glands), from superior to inferior, are the _____, _____, and _____.

6. The three sections of the small intestine beginning with their location proximal to the stomach, are the _____, _____, and _____.

7. The five regions of the large intestine, or _____, beginning proximal to the small intestines are the _____, _____, _____, _____, and _____ portions.

8. Exocrine cell clusters of the pancreas called _____ produce inactive enzymes called _____ as well as active enzymes that are transported to the _____ by way of the _____ and _____ _____ ducts.

9. The three major hormones that control digestion are _____, _____, and _____.

10. A _____ _____ is a protrusion of the upper part of the stomach into the thorax, while a _____ _____ is a protrusion of the small intestine into the pelvic muscles.

Matching

Match each of the following terms with the clue that best describes it by placing the letter of the term in the blank next to the correct clue.

a) buccal

b) cardiac

c) chief cells

d) chyme

e) diverticulosis

f) dysphagia

g) hepatocytes

h) ileocecal valve

i) palate

j) paneth cells

k) parotid

l) peristalsis

m) pyloric

n) sublingual

o) villi

_____ lower stomach sphincter muscle

_____ separates the small and large intestines

_____ associated with the cheeks

_____ moves food through digestive tract

_____ projections of the small-intestine mucosa

_____ salivary gland anterior to the ear

_____ difficult or painful swallowing

_____ lower esophageal sphincter muscle

_____ salivary gland beneath the tongue

_____ leaves the stomach

_____ produce digestive enzymes in the stomach

_____ liver cells

_____ large intestine pocket formation

_____ roof of the mouth

_____ produce antibacterial enzymes

Complete the Terms Table

Complete the missing key terms and/or definitions in the following table.

Term	Definition
	a layer of connective tissue underneath the epithelium of mucosa
	secretory cells of the stomach that produce hydrochloric acid
microvilli	
mesentery	
	absorptive cells of the small intestine
ingestion	
	taken into the body but bypassing the digestive tract
salivary amylase	
enterokinase	
	condition due to a combination of esophageal and gastric reflux
	protistan infection that produces extreme abdominal cramping and chronic diarrhea
cirrhosis	
	excessive bacterial gas production in the large intestine
faliciform ligament	
	a region of the hypothalamus that signals a person has eaten

Label the Graphic

Identify each of the following terms in the illustrations on page 145. Write the number of the anatomical part on the line pointing to its location.

Figure 1 Terms
1. body
2. cardiac sphincter
3. circular muscle layer
4. duodenum
5. esophagus
6. fundus
7. gastroesophageal opening
8. longitudinal muscle layer
9. oblique muscle layer
10. pyloric sphincter
11. pylorus
12. rugae

Figure 2 Terms
1. aorta
2. ascending colon
3. cecum
4. descending colon
5. ileocecal valve
6. ileum
7. inferior vena cava
8. rectum
9. sigmoid colon
10. transverse colon
11. vermiform appendix

Figure 1   Figure 2

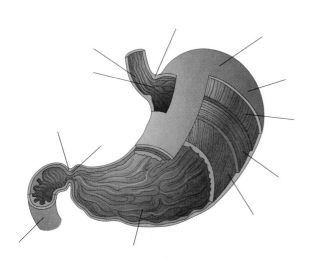   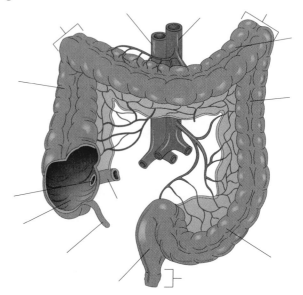

1. What function do the rugae provide for the stomach?

2. In which of the above organs is chyme produced?

3. In which organ does most of the chemical digestion and absorption of nutrients occur?

4. List each muscle or valve identified on the illustrations and specify into what organ it moves the digestive tract contents.

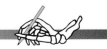

Color the Graphic

Color this illustration using the following color key:

mouth – red
teeth – yellow
salivary glands – pink
pharynx – brown
esophagus – orange
liver – light green
gallbladder – dark green
stomach – light blue
pancreas – purple
small intestine – dark blue
large intestine – black

1. Which digestive system components allow for mastication?

2. The site of digestive enzyme production includes which components?

3. Which component produces bile?

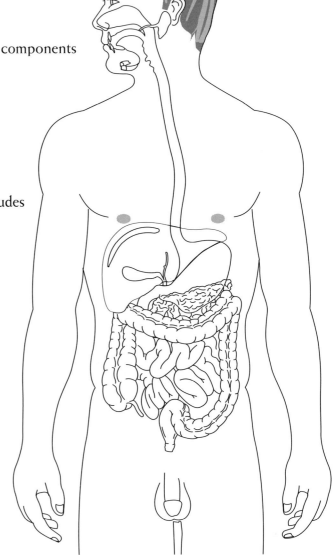

Practical Application

Write brief responses to the following scenarios.

1. Explain the anatomical reasons why ingested food can actually be expelled through the nose or enter into the respiratory passages, rather than entering the esophagus.

2. Describe how surgically blocking off a portion of the stomach aids in weight loss. Discuss how the surgical blockage or removal of a portion of the small intestine would differ in the physiological process contributing to weight loss.

3. What would be the actual cause of the increased flatulence experienced by a person with lactose intolerance as a result of ingesting milk?

4. The hormone changes accompanying pregnancy result in the relaxation of certain smooth muscles in the body. How is this related to the "heartburn" experienced by many women during pregnancy?

5. The presence of fat in chyme stimulates the production of cholecystokinin (CCK). Why would a diet totally void of fat have an effect on the digestion of other nutrients as well?

6. The bacterium *Helicobacter pylori* can penetrate the mucosal lining of the stomach and, in doing so, damages mucous-producing cells. How does this contribute to ulcer formation?

7. Explain the effects that abnormal peristalsis in the colon could have on the digestive system.

8. In which abdominopelvic quadrant would a person experiencing impaction (buildup of fecal matter) in the sigmoid colon experience tenderness? In which quadrant would an individual with gallstones most likely experience tenderness?

9. The genetic disease cystic fibrosis results from a gene that codes for a protein that forms chloride-ion channels. Although the most obvious symptoms of this disease occur in the respiratory system due to abnormal buildup of mucus, the abnormal protein produced by an individual afflicted with this disease also does not allow for proper functioning of certain secretory cells in the pancreas. Secretions produced by affected cells are very thick and viscous. How would this affect the exocrine function of the pancreas?

10. List three ways in which the nervous system is involved in digestive system function.

Crossword Puzzle

Complete the following crossword puzzle using key terms from the text.

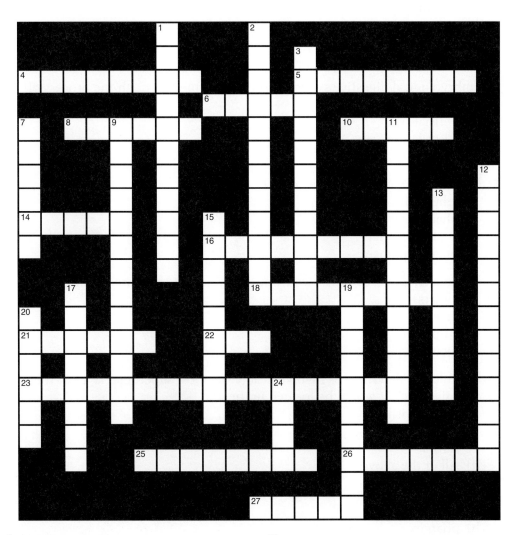

Across

4. watery bowel movements
5. protrudes from the cecum
6. eliminated from colon
8. most posterior molars
10. mucosal erosion
14. projection posterior to the soft palate
16. tongue muscle group attached to bone
18. blood-filled liver cavity
21. terminal portion of the digestive tract
22. peristalsis disorder of unknown cause
23. hunger and thirst are examples of this
25. digests proteins
26. membrane of the tongue
27. lips

Down

1. polyp type that can lead to colon cancer
2. inflammation of the pancreas
3. chewing
7. backflow
9. one of the salivary glands
11. food intolerance of wheat protein
12. lymphatic tissue posterior to the tongue
13. blocks bile flow
15. disease of liver inflammation
17. carry fat to the liver
19. food-poisoning bacteria
20. location of paneth cells
24. digestive tract exit

THE DIGESTIVE SYSTEM

1. Which of the following is not a component of the digestive tract?
   a) mouth
   b) pancreas
   c) stomach
   d) intestines

2. Embryological digestive system tissues are formed through the process of:
   a) blastulation
   b) peristalsis
   c) gastrulation
   d) meiosis

3. Malformation of the tongue could be described as a(n):
   a) lobular disorder
   b) pharyngeal abnormality
   c) uvular disorder
   d) lingual anomaly

4. When a child has lost his "two front teeth," which teeth are missing?
   a) molars
   b) incisors
   c) cuspids
   d) bicuspids

5. If an ulcer is described as involving only the most superficial layer of the digestive tract, it would be located in the:
   a) muscularis layer
   b) mucosa
   c) serosa
   d) All of the above

6. Acid reflux could cause damage to the:
   a) esophagus
   b) pharynx
   c) throat
   d) All of the above

7. Cells in the stomach produce:
   a) hydrochloric acid
   b) proteases
   c) gastrin
   d) All of the above

8. Microvilli are projections on the epithelial cells lining the _____.
   a) small intestine
   b) stomach
   c) large intestine
   d) All of the above

9. Which of the following types of cells would not be found in the small intestine?
   a) paneth cells
   b) enterocytes
   c) enteroendocrine
   d) acini

10. Which of the following is true about zymogens?
    a) They are produced only in the small intestine.
    b) They are active enzymes.
    c) They are transported by the pancreatic and common bile ducts.
    d) All of the above

11. Which of the following best describes the liver?
    a) comprises four lobes
    b) produces bile
    c) is capable of regeneration
    d) All of the above

12. Which of the following is not a function of the liver?
    a) formation of serum globulins
    b) production of digestive enzymes
    c) breakdown of amino acids
    d) synthesis of heparin

13. Diet pills that help control the sensation of hunger would most likely have a direct effect on:
    a) bile production
    b) the colon
    c) the hypothalamus
    d) peristalsis

14. Cholecystokinin stimulates:
    a) pancreatic enzyme production
    b) hydrochloric acid production by the stomach
    c) bicarbonate production by the pancreas
    d) All of the above

15. Which of the following is absorbed in the stomach?
    a) amino acids and lipids
    b) glucose
    c) alcohol and drugs
    d) All of the above

16. The site of most chemical digestion and absorption is the:
    a) small intestine
    b) stomach
    c) large intestine
    d) All of the above

17. Most fluids and electrolytes are transferred from the the digestive tract to the blood stream in the:
    a) small intestine
    b) stomach
    c) large intestine
    d) All of the above

18. Which of the following is not true of the hepatic-portal system?
    a) It transfers bile to the small intestine.
    b) It allows absorbed nutrients to be further "processed" before entering general circulation.
    c) It transports blood from the digestive tract to the liver.
    d) It allows removal of many toxic substances.

19. The bicarbonate component of pancreatic fluid:
    a) chemically digests food
    b) is produced in response to CCK
    c) increases the pH of chyme
    d) All of the above

20. Which of the following is true of *Salmonella?*
    a) is linked to ulcer formation
    b) is a protozoan
    c) can cause inflammatory bowel disease
    d) is a common cause of food poisoning

21. A scar resulting from an appendectomy (removal of the appendix) would be found:
    a) in the upper right quadrant
    b) in the lower right quadrant
    c) in the upper left quadrant
    d) in the lower left quadrant

22. Colon polyps are:
    a) not a very common disorder
    b) often associated with diets high in fat and low in fiber
    c) always considered to be a serious health threat
    d) All of the above

23. The segment of the colon located between the hepatic and splenic flexure is the:
    a) descending
    b) ascending
    c) sigmoid
    d) transverse

24. Starch digestion begins in the:
    a) stomach
    b) mouth
    c) duodenum
    d) jejunum

25. Age-related decline in liver and gallbladder function results in decreased digestion of:
    a) proteins
    b) starches
    c) fats
    d) All of the above

CHAPTER

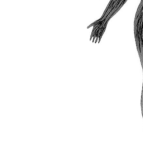

14

THE URINARY SYSTEM

Completion

Complete the following sentences by filling in each blank with a key term from the text.

1. The _____ are the organs that actually form urine, while the _____, _____ _____, and _____ are the organs and structures that form the conduction system that carries it out of the body.

2. Each kidney is surrounded by a cushion of fat called the _____ _____. It is secured to the abdominal wall by a connective-tissue covering called the _____ _____, and it has a concave indentation known as the _____, which is the entry point for the _____ _____ and the exit for the _____ _____ and _____.

3. Within the kidneys, urine is formed in the microscopic physiological units called _____, and is transported to the internal storage cavity of the kidneys, or _____ _____, through extensions called _____.

4. The nephron is composed of _____ _____ that expand to form _____ _____. Within the capsule is the folded capillary called the _____. The structure formed by the latter two components is called the _____ _____.

5. The nephron tubular arrangement has four major segments: 1) the _____ _____ _____; 2) the _____ _____ _____; 3) the _____ _____ _____; and 4) the _____ _____.

6. Urine formation can be thought of as a three-step process: 1) _____ _____; 2) _____ _____; and 3) _____ _____.

153

7. Most reabsorption occurs in the proximal convoluted tubule by a combination of _____ _____ (osmosis and facilitated diffusion) and _____ _____ (pumping).

8. The transfer of many ions from the blood stream into the _____ through the process of _____ _____ helps to maintain a desirable body fluid pH.

9. _____ _____ and _____ are both hormones that aid in water retention in the renal tubules, while the hormone _____ _____ _____ causes diuresis.

10. Swelling of the glomerular membranes is known as _____. It can be categorized on the basis of symptoms as being a urinary system disorder of _____, or based on etiology as an _____ disorder.

Matching

Match each of the following terms with the clue that best describes it by placing the letter of the term in the blank next to the correct clue.

a) anuria   _____ water excretion from the body

b) caliculi   _____ collected in the renal corpuscle

c) diuresis   _____ moved by carrier proteins

d) external urethral sphincter   _____ body exit for urine

e) filtrate   _____ triangular-shaped medulla tissue

f) hemodialysis   _____ voluntary muscular ring

g) internal urinary sphincter   _____ kidney stones

h) micturition   _____ urine voiding

i) polyuria   _____ behind the abdominal cavity lining

j) renal columns   _____ reabsorption in the collecting tube

k) renal pyramids   _____ excess urine production

l) retroperitoneal   _____ extensions of the cortex

m) symported   _____ artificial blood-filtering procedure

n) urethral orifice   _____ involuntary muscular ring

o) water conservation _____ lack of urine production

Complete the Terms Table

Complete the missing key terms and/or definitions in the following table.

Term	Definition
	a capillary loop within the nephron
	loss of the voluntary control of holding urine in the bladder
urinary retention	
	abnormal loss of fluid from the body
urine concentration	
	the process by which plasma and many dissolved substances are moved from the blood into Bowman's capsule
tubular reabsorption	
	the process by which certain waste products and ions are removed from the blood into the tubular fluid
	hormone secreted by special cardiac cells that functions to lower blood volume and blood pressure
polycystic kidney disease	
	irreparable nephron damage and loss of kidney function
cystocele	

Label the Graphic

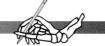

Identify each of the following terms in the illustrations on page 156. Write the number of the anatomical part on the line(s) pointing to its location.

1. abdominal aorta
2. adrenal glands
3. calyces
4. cortex
5. external urinary meatus (orifice)
6. inferior vena cava
7. left kidney
8. medulla (renal pyramid)
9. pelvis
10. renal artery
11. renal vein
12. right kidney
13. ureter
14. urethra
15. urinary bladder

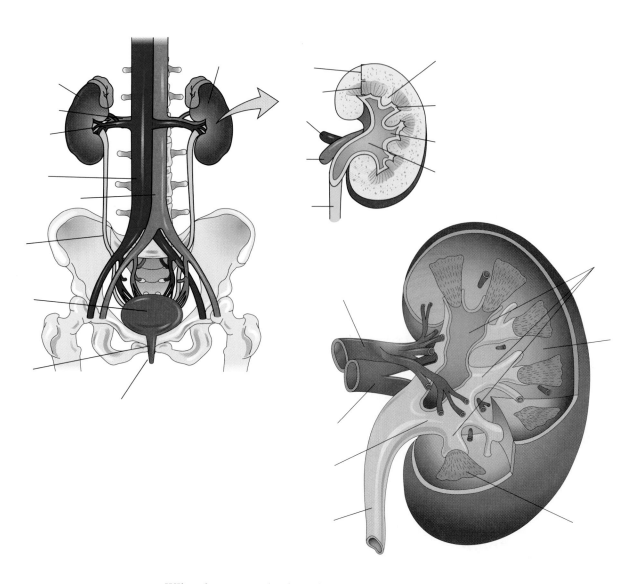

1. What hormone do the adrenal glands produce that influences urine formation?

2. Through which of the illustrated blood vessels does blood that has been filtered by the kidneys return to the heart?

3. Through which of the illustrated blood vessels is blood that is to be filtered by the kidneys carried?

Color the Graphic

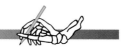

Color this illustration using the following color key:

arteries – red
veins – blue
glomerulus – pink
Bowman's capsule – yellow
proximal convoluted tubule – orange
descending loop of Henle – light green
ascending loop of Henle – dark green
distal convoluted tubule – brown
collecting tubule – black

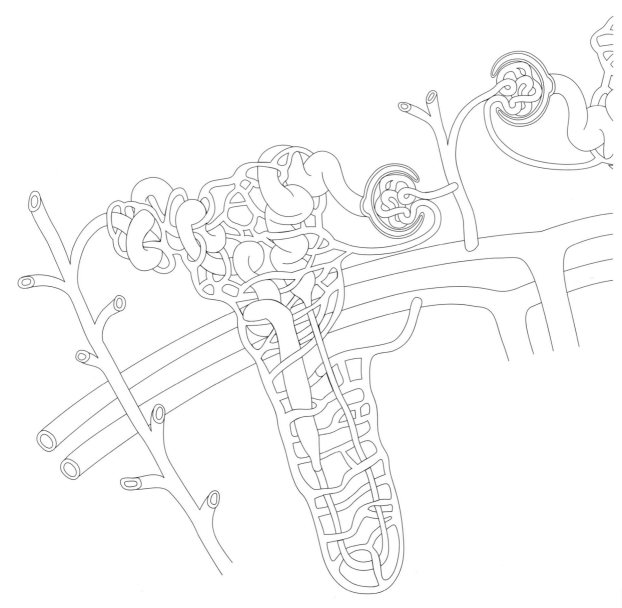

THE URINARY SYSTEM

1. What two structures illustrated are the structural components of the renal corpuscle?

2. What physiological step of urine formation occurs in the renal corpuscle?

3. What physiological steps of urine formation occur in all areas of the peritubular capillary system?

4. In what structure does the majority of urine concentration occur?

Practical Application

Write brief responses to the following scenarios.

1. Describe one way in which the urinary system would affect the pH regulation of the respiratory system.

2. Briefly discuss one way in which the urinary system has an effect on the circulatory system.

3. Since the influence of one organ system over another is usually a reciprocal relationship, briefly discuss one way in which the circulatory system directly affects the urinary system.

4. Can you think of any role that the skeletal system plays in the urinary system?

5. The text discusses in some detail the role that the endocrine system plays in urinary system function, but can you think of a way that the urinary system provides for the endocrine system?

6. Explain why the abnormal protein loss through the body surface of patients suffering from severe burns contributes to edema and dehydration.

7. How does the anatomical location of the ureter-bladder connection point aid in the ability of the bladder to act as a reservoir for urine?

8. How would hyperkalemia (high blood-potassium levels) influence diuresis?

9. Specific gravity is a measurement that indicates the density of a fluid compared with that of water. Water is said to have a specific gravity of 1. Any addition of solute will increase the specific gravity. Because urine is not pure water, but contains many dissolved substances, its normal specific gravity is greater than 1. What effect would a decrease in ADH have on diuresis, and how would this affect the specific gravity of urine?

10. Why is a hypertensive patient encouraged to restrict consumption?

159

Crossword Puzzle

Complete the following crossword puzzle using key terms from the text.

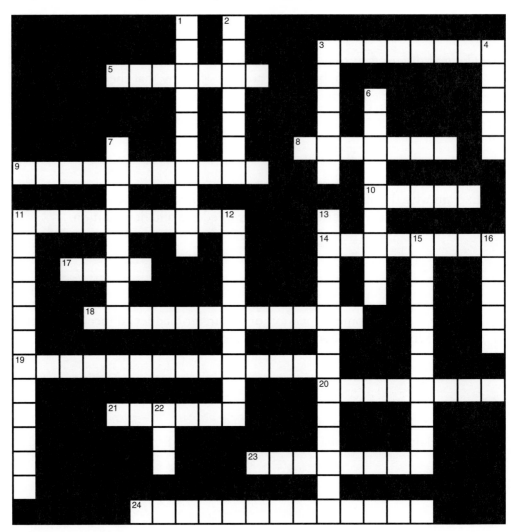

Across

3. drainage tube
5. painful urination
8. inner kidney tissue
9. elevated urine protein
10. tissue fluid retention
11. renal calculus
14. decreased urine production
17. aggregate of cells in urine
18. epithelial lining of the bladder
19. nephron inflammation
20. inflammation of the renal pelvis
21. indication of UTI
23. bladder inflammation
24. presence of urinary amino acids

Down

1. presence of urinary glucose
2. located on the bladder floor
3. outer kidney tissue
4. inward folds
6. chemicals that increase urine water
7. bladder smooth muscle
11. floating kidney
12. blood in the urine
13. symported
15. urethral inflammation
16. temporary renal failure
22. short for urinary tract infection

Quiz

1. Which of the following is not a function of the urinary system?

   a) maintenance of body pH
   b) electrolyte balance
   c) immune regulation
   d) osmotic homeostasis

2. The ureters and urethra:
   a) alter the urine composition
   b) reabsorb water
   c) conduct urine
   d) All of the above

3. The renal pyramids are:
   a) located in the renal medulla
   b) the location of urine collection tubules
   c) separated by renal columns
   d) All of the above

4. Which of the following is the correct sequence of urine transfer out of the kidney?
   a) calyces, collecting duct, renal pelvis, ureter
   b) collecting duct, calyces, renal pelvis, ureter
   c) renal pelvis, collecting duct, calyces, ureter
   d) collecting duct, renal pelvis, calyces, ureter

5. Voluntary control of micturition is provided by:
   a) the internal urinary sphincter
   b) the urethral orifice
   c) the external urinary sphincter
   d) All of the above

6. The urinary bladder has the ability to distend and act as a urine reservoir because of:
   a) the arrangement of the detrusor muscle fibers
   b) the transitional epithelial lining
   c) involuntary closure of the internal urinary sphincter
   d) All of the above

7. Females are more susceptible to bacterial urinary tract infections than are males due to:
   a) hormonal differences
   b) smaller bladder size
   c) length and location of the urethra
   d) All of the above

8. Which of the following is not a term referring to abnormal urine production?
   a) polyuria
   b) urinary retention
   c) anuria
   d) None of the above

9. Blood is carried to the glomerulus by the:
   a) efferent arteriole
   b) afferent arteriole
   c) renal artery
   d) renal vein

10. Which of the following is true of the peritubular capillary system?
    a) It consists of the glomerulus and Bowman's capsule.
    b) It is the site of urine filtration.
    c) It is the part of the nephron distal to the renal corpuscle.
    d) All of the above

11. Which of the following is a correct sequence of the tubular arrangement within the nephron?
    a) Bowman's capsule, proximal convoluted tubules, loop of Henle
    b) proximal convoluted tubules, loop of Henle, distal convoluted tubules
    c) loop of Henle, distal convoluted tubules, collecting duct
    d) All of the above

12. Urine filtration occurs in the:
    a) renal corpuscle
    b) afferent arteriole
    c) loop of Henle
    d) collecting duct

13. Tubular reabsorption:
    a) occurs in the peritubular capillary system
    b) returns water, nutrients, and electrolytes to the blood
    c) is under some hormonal influence
    d) All of the above

14. Which of the following is not a true statement about tubular secretion?
    a) It removes waste products from the blood.
    b) It aids in homeostasis of body pH.
    c) It elevates blood glucose levels.
    d) It contributes to urine electrolyte levels.

15. Urine concentration occurs in which part of the nephron?
    a) glomerulus
    b) proximal convoluted tubule
    c) collecting duct
    d) All of the above

16. Water moves out of the collecting duct due to:
    a) the action of antidiuretic hormone on its wall permeability
    b) the concentration gradient that exists between the tubular fluid and the interstitial fluid of the kidney medulla
    c) osmosis
    d) All of the above

17. High blood-potassium levels would stimulate the production of:
    a) antidiuretic hormone
    b) aldosterone
    c) atrial natriuretic factor
    d) angiotensin II

18. Which of the following hormones does not exert its effect on the nephron peritubular system?
    a) antidiuretic hormone
    b) aldosterone
    c) atrial natriuretic factor
    d) angiotensin II

19. Which of the following hormones would increase the water content of the urine?
    a) antidiuretic hormone
    b) aldosterone
    c) atrial natriuretic factor
    d) angiotensin II

20. Which of the following categories of urinary system diseases would not apply to polycystic kidney disease?
    a) infection
    b) genetic
    c) congenital
    d) degenerative

21. Which of the following types of inflammation does not occur in the conduction system components of the urinary system?
    a) cystitis
    b) urethritis
    c) pyelitis
    d) pyelonephritis

22. The presence of both proteinuria and hematuria may be indicative of:
    a) dysuria
    b) edema
    c) glomerulonephritis
    d) All of the above

23. Glucosuria and aminoaciduria:
    a) may lead to the formation of kidney or bladder calculi
    b) indicate normal urine values
    c) always indicate deficiency of these nutrients
    d) have no effect on the osmolarity of the filtrate

24. Most malignancies in the urinary system:
    a) are fatal despite early detection
    b) produce symptoms uncommon to other urinary system disorders
    c) require imaging techniques for definitive diagnosis
    d) All of the above

25. Most effects of urinary system aging are:
    a) the result of nephron function loss
    b) unrelated to the function of other body systems
    c) related to the coinciding increased incidence of disease
    d) All of the above

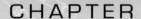

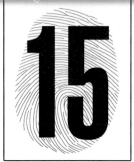

15 THE REPRODUCTIVE SYSTEM AND HUMAN DEVELOPMENT

Completion

Complete the following sentences by filling in each blank with a key term from the text.

1. Human sexual reproductive organs called _____ contain mobile cells called _____ _____ _____.

2. The organs of the female reproductive system that produce and transport the egg and developed fetus comprise the _____ _____ which consists of the _____, _____ _____, _____, and _____.

3. The inner layer of the uterus is a thick mucosa called the _____, which is shed during a period called the _____ _____.

4. The external genitalia of the female are collectively known as the _____ which consist of the fat pad covering the pubic bone called the _____, the outer "lips" called the _____ _____, and the inner "lips" or _____ _____, which protect the sensitive erectile tissue known as the _____.

5. In the male the internal network of tubes and glands that assist with the transport of sperm is called the _____ _____, while the external genitalia consist of the _____ and _____.

6. Sperm maturation and storage occur in the _____ until the sperm are expelled into the _____ _____, where they mix with the fluid containing enzymes, fructose, hormones, lipids, and proteins which are produced by the _____ _____ that facilitate their survival. The mixture of sperm and this fluid is called _____, which is transferred to the vagina during sexual intercourse in the ejection process known as _____.

7. Blood enters the penis through the _____ _____ to enter the inner sheath of erectile tissue called the _____ _____, which prevents the urethra from closing the two outer chambers of erectile tissue called the _____ _____, which causes the penile enlargement and hardening known as _____.

8. The female sexual cycle, or _____ _____, can actually be thought of as two cycles based on the major organs involved: the _____ and _____. The first prepares the egg for fertilization and can be further divided into the _____ and _____ phases, while the second involves the _____ _____, in which the endometrium thickens to prepare for pregnancy.

9. A fertilized egg is called a(n) _____. It divides to become a _____ as it travels down the fallopian tube to the uterus where _____, or its attachment to the endometrium, occurs. This induces the development of the nourishing organ called the _____. It then develops into a _____ where differentiation of tissues occurs. This is followed by continued growth until it finally becomes known as a _____.

10. Location of the placenta in the lower part of the uterus is a condition known as _____ _____, which blocks the route of normal birth and usually requires surgical removal of the baby through the abdominal wall, or a(n) _____ _____.

Matching

Match each of the following terms with the clue that best describes it by placing the letter of the term in the blank next to the correct clue.

a) androgen

b) circumcision

c) copulation

d) Cowper's glands

e) ectopic

f) fimbriae

g) glans

h) lactation

i) oocyte

j) ovary

k) ovum

l) perineum

m) prostate gland

n) seminiferous tubules

o) testis

_____ milk production

_____ immature egg

_____ produces the mucus-like component of semen

_____ female gonad

_____ the tip of the penis

_____ produces the alkaline component of semen

_____ site of sperm production in the testes

_____ finger-like oviduct projections

_____ surgical removal of the penis foreskin

_____ male gonad

_____ sexual intercourse

_____ development of secondary male sex characteristics

_____ pregnancy outside of the uterus

_____ external area of the pelvic floor

_____ mature egg

165

Complete the Terms Table

Complete the missing key terms and/or definitions in the following table.

Term	Definition
	developmental differences that distinguish the two genders
external genitalia	
	a fluid-filled sac in which an egg matures
corpus luteum	
	a condition in which it is not clear at birth whether the individual is a male or a female
lactiferous ducts	
	cells that produce testosterone in the testis
menses	
	an intense sensation that occurs at the height of sexual excitement
conception	
	a hormone produced by the placenta that maintains pregnancy; it is triggered by the release of estrogen and progesterone
	a fluid-filled sac that surrounds the fetus
hypospadia	
	cessation of the menstrual periods
andropause	

Label the Graphic

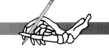

Identify each of the following terms in the illustration on page 167. Write the number of the anatomical part on the line pointing to its location.

Figure 1 Terms
1. body of the uterus
2. cervix
3. fallopian tube
4. fundus of uterus
5. ovary
6. pubic bone
7. rectum
8. ureter
9. urethra
10. urinary bladder
11. vagina

Figure 2 Terms
1. anus
2. Cowper's (bulbourethral) gland
3. ductus (vas) deferens
4. epididymis
5. penis prostate gland
6. rectum
7. scrotum
8. seminal vesicle
9. testis
10. ureter
11. urethra
12. urinary bladder

Figure 1   Figure 2

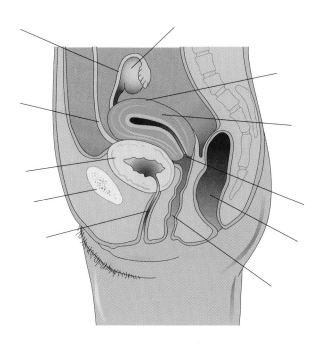

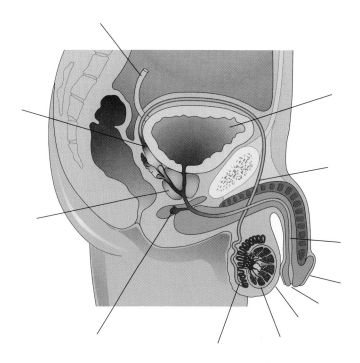

1. What structure carries the egg to the uterus?

2. Where does implantation normally take place?

3. Where are sperm produced?

4. What is the site of maturation and storage of sperm?

THE REPRODUCTIVE SYSTEM AND HUMAN DEVELOPMENT

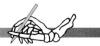

Color this illustration using the following color key:

blastula entering uterus – light green
blastula implanting – dark green
embryo – purple
endometrium of uterine wall – pink
fallopian tube – yellow
fertilization – green
ovary – outline in black
ovulated egg – orange
uterine muscle wall – brown
zygote – blue

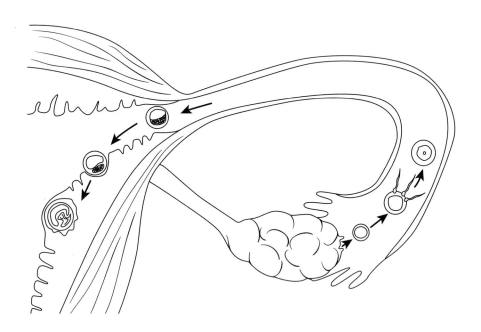

1. What is the name given to the stage of embryo tissue differentiation?

2. By what term is the developing embryo identified in the most advanced stages prior to birth?

Practical Application

Write brief responses to the following scenarios.

1. Describe the pathway that sperm travel from their site of production through their exit from the body during ejaculation in reference to other anatomical organs and structures of the male reproductive and urinary systems.

2. What is significant about the anatomy of the female reproductive tract that could actually allow bacterial infection of the abdominal cavity?

3. List two enzymatic or hormonal abnormalities in a female that could result in the development of male secondary sex characteristics.

4. Explain the physiological reason that wearing tight fitting underwear could contribute to a low sperm count in a male.

5. What effect could an abnormally high level of estrogen or testosterone in a pregnant female have on the developing fetus?

6. How are ectopic and tubal pregnancies possible?

7. Erectile dysfunction can occur from improper neural stimulation. Which division of the nervous system is involved in this disorder, and how does it cause the inability to obtain an erection?

8. What role do the breasts play in reproduction?

9. Would a vasectomy or tubal ligation (surgical interruption of the fallopian tube pathway) have any effect on normal hormone production or gamete formation?

10. Using your knowledge of the female menstrual cycle explain the mathematics behind the statistic that females produce 350 to 500 ova throughout a normal life span.

Crossword Puzzle

Complete the following crossword puzzle using key terms from the text.

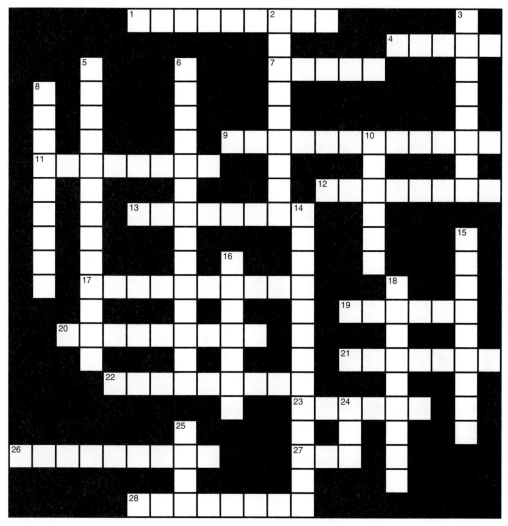

Across

1. twins developed from one egg
4. membrane covering the vaginal opening
7. onset of childbirth
9. loss of an erection
11. fallopian tubes
12. blood-filling tissue
13. enzyme packet in head of sperm
17. cancer of the testes
19. cancer of the mammary glands
20. twins whose bodies are joined together
21. milk-producing glands
22. converts androgens into estrogen
23. center of mammary gland
26. egg release from the ovary
27. genital warts is an example of this
28. noncancerous uterine tumors

Down

2. initial mammary gland product
3. cancer of the uterine opening to the vagina
5. egg and sperm fusion
6. undescended testis
8. anatomical visual sex characteristics
10. mucous-producing urethral glands
14. process of embryo formation
15. twins developed from two eggs
16. stage of sexual maturation
18. converts cholesterol to progesterone
24. a common cause of female infertility
25. uterus

THE REPRODUCTIVE SYSTEM AND HUMAN DEVELOPMENT

1. Which of the following is not related to puberty?
   a) development of secondary sex characteristics
   b) sexual dimorphism
   c) differentiation of gonads
   d) sexual reproductive capability

2. Mammary glands:
   a) are present only in females
   b) depend on estrogen for growth and development
   c) are considered to be primary sex organs
   d) All of the above

3. The ovaries:
   a) are the site of egg production
   b) are attached to the fallopian tubes
   c) are located adjacent to the kidneys
   d) All of the above

4. Which of the following is not a true statement concerning egg production?
   a) ova (plural for ovum) are present at birth
   b) ova are produced through meiosis of oocytes
   c) oocytes are contained within ovarian follicles
   d) ovulation is the release of an ovum from a graafian follicle

5. Which of the following is a true statement concerning the corpus luteum?
   a) It is active in the ovarian follicular stage.
   b) It is formed prior to ovulation.
   c) It produces progesterone.
   d) All of the above

6. The fallopian tubes:
   a) are the site of fertilization
   b) are held in place by the broad ligament
   c) function for peristalsis by contraction of the myosalpinx
   d) All of the above

7. Which of the following is a true statement about the anatomy of the uterus?
   a) It contains the myometriuman, outer muscular layer.
   b) It contains the endometrium, an inner mucosal layer.
   c) It is connected to the vagina at the cervix.
   d) All of the above

8. Which of the following is not a component of the external female genitalia?
   a) labia minora
   b) mons
   c) vagina
   d) clitoris

9. The testes contain the:
    a) seminal vesicles
    b) epididymis
    c) seminiferous tubules
    d) All of the above

10. The seminal vessels include the:
    a) vas deferens
    b) seminal vesicles
    c) prostate gland
    d) All of the above

11. Which of the following is not a component of the male external genitalia?
    a) Cowper's gland
    b) scrotum
    c) penis
    d) phallus

12. The most internal component of the penis is the:
    a) glans
    b) urethra
    c) foreskin
    d) corpus cavernosum

13. The ovarian cycle:
    a) leads to ovulation
    b) is divided into follicular and luteal stages
    c) includes development of the corpus luteum
    d) All of the above

14. The proliferative stage of the menstrual cycle:
    a) occurs only following pregnancy
    b) precedes the ovarian cycle
    c) produces a thickened endometrium
    d) All of the above

15. Erection of the penis results from:
    a) sympathetic innervation
    b) contriction of arteries and dilation of veins
    c) contriction of veins and dilation of arteries
    d) decreased parasympathetic innervation

16. Which of the following is not a true statement regarding components of semen?
    a) It contains sperm produced in the testes.
    b) It contains nutrients, hormones, and enzymes produced by the seminal vesicles.
    c) It contains an alkaline substance produced by the prostate gland.
    d) All of the above

173

17. Which of the following is the correct normal functioning sequence of events for males during copulation?
    a) sexual arousal, erection, ejaculation, detumescence
    b) detumescence, erection, sexual arousal, ejaculation
    c) sexual arousal, detumescence, erection, ejaculation
    d) sexual arousal, detumescence, erection, ejaculation

18. Which of the following is a normal female sexual response?
    a) erectile tissue response of the clitoris and nipples
    b) mucous production by Skene's glands
    c) muscle contractions of the vaginal tract and cervix
    d) All of the above

19. Penetration of the egg by sperm is made possible by:
    a) the acidic pH of the vagina
    b) the sperm flagella
    c) enzymes contained in the sperm structure called the acrosome
    d) the corpus luteum

20. At the point of implantation the developing fertilized egg is called:
    a) zygote
    b) gastrula
    c) blastula
    d) fetus

21. Formation of the placenta:
    a) is initiated by implantation
    b) marks the true state of pregnancy
    c) allows for nourishment of the developing embryo
    d) All of the above

22. What hormone has a similar structure to pollutants thought to have a detrimental effect on normal male embryological development?
    a) androgen
    b) estrogen
    c) progesterone
    d) testosterone

23. Sexually-transmitted diseases can be spread through:
    a) copulation
    b) infectious viruses, bacteria, or protistans
    c) oral and anal sex
    d) All of the above

24. Which of the following is not a disorder associated with pregnancy?
    a) fibroids
    b) placenta previa
    c) ectopic implantation
    d) All of the above

25. Age-related changes in the reproductive system:
    a) usually have no effect on sexual function
    b) always decrease the sex drive
    c) are most commonly associated with changes in the endocrine and urinary systems
    d) All of the above